AF147570

Clinicians' Guides to Radionuclide Hybrid Imaging

PET/CT

Series Editors

Jamshed B. Bomanji, Nuclear Medicine, University College Hospital
London, UK

Gopinath Gnanasegaran, Department of Nuclear Medicine
Royal Free London NHS Foundation Trust, London, UK

Stefano Fanti, Deptartment of Nuclear Medicine
Policlinico S.Orsola-Malpighi, Bologna, Bologna, Italy

Homer A. Macapinlac, Department of Nuclear Medicine
The University of Texas MD Anderson Cancer Center, Houston, TX, USA

Hybrid imaging with PET/CT and SPECT/CT provides high-quality information on function and structure, thereby permitting accurate localization, characterization, and diagnosis. There is extensive evidence to support the value of PET/CT, which has made a significant impact on oncological imaging and the management of patients with cancer. The evidence in favor of SPECT/CT, especially for orthopaedic indications, is evolving and increasing. This pocket book series on hybrid imaging (PET/CT and SPECT/CT) is specifically aimed at referring clinicians, nuclear medicine/radiology physicians, radiographers/technologists, and nurses who routinely work in nuclear medicine and participate in multidisciplinary meetings. The series will include 18 pocket books on PET/CT and 3 on SPECT/CT. Compiled under the auspices of the British Nuclear Medicine Society, the series is the joint work of many colleagues and professionals worldwide who share a common vision and purpose in promoting and supporting nuclear medicine as an important imaging specialty for the diagnosis and management of oncological and non-oncological conditions.

The PET/CT pocket book series will be dedicated to some of the Society's recently departed peers, including Prof Ignac Fogelman, Dr Muriel Buxton-Thomas and Prof Ajit K Padhy

More information about this series at http://www.springer.com/series/13803

Rakesh Kumar • Kanhaiyalal Agrawal
Narainder K. Gupta
Editors

PET/CT in Breast Cancer

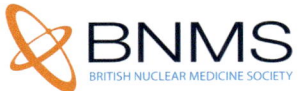

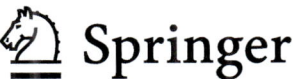

Editors
Rakesh Kumar
Department of Nuclear Medicine
All India Institute of Medical Sciences
New Delhi, Delhi, India

Kanhaiyalal Agrawal
Department of Nuclear Medicine
All India Institute of Medical Sciences
Bhubaneswar, Odisha, India

Narainder K. Gupta
Department of Radiology
Hospital of the University of Pennsylvania
Philadelphia, PA, USA

ISSN 2367-2439   ISSN 2367-2447   (electronic)
PET/CT
ISBN 978-3-031-29589-8   ISBN 978-3-031-29590-4   (eBook)
https://doi.org/10.1007/978-3-031-29590-4

This Springer imprint is published by the registered company Springer Nature Switzerland AG
The registered company address is: Gewerbestrasse 11, 6330 Cham, Switzerland

The PET/CT pocket book series will be dedicated to some of the Society's recently departed peers, including Prof Ignac Fogelman, Dr Muriel Buxton-Thomas and Prof Ajit K Padhy.

Foreword

Clear and concise clinical indications for PET/CT in the management of the oncology patient are presented in this series of 20 separate booklets. The impact on better staging, tailored management and specific treatment of the patient with cancer has been achieved with the advent of this multimodality imaging technology. Early and accurate diagnosis will always pay, and clear information can be gathered with PET/CT on treatment responses. Prognostic information is gathered and can forward guide additional therapeutic options.

It is a fortunate coincidence that PET/CT was able to derive great benefit from radionuclide-labelled probes, which deliver good and often excellent target to non-target signals. Whilst labelled glucose remains the cornerstone for the clinical benefit achieved, a number of recent probes are definitely adding benefit. PET/CT is hence an evolving technology, extending its applications and indications. Significant advances in the instrumentation and data processing available have also contributed to this technology, which delivers high-throughput and a wealth of data, with good patient tolerance and indeed patient and public acceptance. As an example, the role of PET/CT in the evaluation of cardiac disease is also covered, with an emphasis on labelled rubidium and labelled glucose studies.

The novel probes of labelled choline, labelled peptides, such as DOTATATE, and, most recently, labelled PSMA (prostate-specific membrane antigen) have gained rapid clinical utility and acceptance, as significant PET/CT tools for the management of neuroendocrine disease and prostate cancer patients, notwithstanding all the advances achieved with other imaging modalities, such as MRI. Hence, a chapter reviewing novel PET tracers forms part of this series.

The oncological community has recognised the value of PET/CT and has delivered advanced diagnostic criteria for some of the most important indications for PET/CT. This includes the recent Deauville criteria for the classification of PET/CT patients with lymphoma—similar criteria are expected to develop for other malignancies, such as head and neck cancer, melanoma and pelvic malignancies. For completion, a separate section covers the role of PET/CT in radiotherapy planning, discussing the indications for planning biological tumour volumes in relevant cancers.

These booklets offer simple, rapid and concise guidelines on the utility of PET/CT in a range of oncological indications. They also deliver a rapid aide memoire on the merits and appropriate indications for PET/CT in oncology.

London, UK   Peter J. Ell

Preface

As the use of PET/CT in oncology is expanding, it is essential for *Nuclear Medicine* and related oncology professionals to continuously update their knowledge. The main aim of this book is to provide crisp information related to pathology, management and radiological/molecular imaging in breast carcinoma. In this book, we have mentioned the concise information on pathology, management and radiological/molecular imaging in breast carcinoma along with detailed information on FDG PET/CT in breast cancer, normal variants, artefacts, pitfalls with atlas illustrations. The chapters are written by pathologist, oncologist, radiologist and Nuclear Medicine experts from different countries with enormous experience in breast cancer practice. The book is unique in providing quick reference to practice of PET/CT in breast cancer. The intended readers are mostly nuclear medicine physicians and radiologists, but it may be of interest to wider medical community including oncologist and radiotherapist.

We are extremely grateful to the BNMS Education Committee, the BNMS council members and series editors for their enthusiasm and trust. We want to thank all those people who have contributed to this work as advisors, authors and reviewers, without whom the book would not have been possible.

New Delhi, India   Rakesh Kumar
Bhubaneswar, India   Kanhaiyalal Agrawal
Philadelphia, PA, USA   Narainder K. Gupta

Acknowledgements

The series co-ordinators and editors would like to express sincere gratitude to the members of the British Nuclear Medicine Society, patients, teachers, colleagues, students, the industry and the BNMS Education Committee Members for their continued support and inspiration.

Andy Bradley
Brent Drake
Francis Sundram
James Ballinger
Parthiban Arumugam
Rizwan Syed
Sai Han
Vineet Prakash

Contents

Clinical Background of Breast Cancer

1

Charlie Zhou and Siraj Yusuf

Contents

1.1 Epidemiology and Risk Factors

Breast cancer is the most common cancer by incidence worldwide with approximately 2.4 million new cases diagnosed every year [1]. It is the leading oncological cause of death amongst women and the fifth leading oncological cause of death overall, responsible for 534,000 death per annum worldwide. The burden of disease falls disproportionately on higher-income countries, where lifetime risk of breast cancer among women is 1 in 9. Overall, age-standardized incidence and death rates are approximately four- and twofold higher, respectively, in North America, Western Europe, and Australia in comparison to East Asia, South Asia, and Latin America. However, observed breast cancer incidence appears to be rising in developing countries while they have largely plateaued in more developed nations [2].

C. Zhou (✉)
Royal Free London NHS Foundation Trust, London, UK
e-mail: Charlie.zhou@doctors.org.uk

S. Yusuf
Nuclear Medicine and Radiology, The Royal Marsden NHS Foundation Trust, London, UK

Breast cancer is caused by a complex interplay between genetic and environmental factors. There is a strong preponderance based on gender, with incidence in women occurring 50–100 fold more frequently than in men [1]. As with all malignant diseases, the risk of breast cancer increases greatly with age. It occurs less frequently in women under the age of 40 years, and the risk of breast cancer increases steadily following menopause [3].

Approximately 5–10% of incident cases can be attributed to a genetic driver. The best-described genetic predispositions are mutations involving the BRCA 1 and BRCA 2 tumor suppressor genes, where lifetime risk of breast cancer approaches 65% [4]. A number of other mutations have also been implicated in breast cancer risk, and have been predominantly implicated in DNA repair pathways and cell cycle control. Other non-modifiable risk factors include increasing height and Caucasian ethnicity.

Lifelong exposures to sex hormones and estrogen, in particular, have been strongly associated with breast cancer [5]. A range of other factors including early menarche, late menopause, low parity, obesity, and treatment with the oral contraceptive pill or hormone replacement therapy have also been observed to have higher than expected rates of breast cancer (Table 1.1). In addition, male breast cancer risk is also associated with factors that may increase estrogen exposure including liver disease, Klinefelter syndrome, or exogenous sex hormone therapy.

A number of modifiable risk factors have also been identified, including alcohol consumption, smoking, a high-fat diet, as well as shift work. Previous exposure to radiation and certain occupational chemicals has also been implicated in breast cancer risk.

Table 1.1 Risk factors for breast cancer

Non-modifiable
Sex
Age
Genetic predisposition
Height
Ethnicity
Modifiable
Alcohol
Smoking
Diet
Shift work
Occupational exposure
Hormonal
Early menarche
Late menopause
Low parity
Oral contraceptive pill
Hormonal replacement therapy
Obesity
Liver disease

1.1.1 Clinical Presentation

The most common presentation of breast cancer is the finding of a new breast lump (although it should be noted that more than 80% of breast lumps are eventually found to be benign). However, any noticeable change in the architecture of the breast such as change in size or shape, thickening of the breast tissue, dimpling or tethering of the skin or new inversion of the nipple, should warrant consideration of underlying malignancy. Inflammatory breast cancer may manifest in the absence of a discrete tissue mass.

Certain reported clinical manifestations should elicit a higher index of suspicion for malignancy. *Peau d'orange* occurs when malignancy-induced cutaneous lymphatic edema causes localized swelling of the breast but the inelastic Cooper ligaments of the breast tether the overlying skin, resulting in a dimpled appearance akin to the skin of an orange. Paget's disease of the nipple is characterized by a local eczematous change in the periareolar skin, which may be associated with discharge, altered sensation, and nipple inversion. Although commonly misconstrued as a purely benign condition, it may be associated with underlying malignancy and can result in delayed diagnosis.

Patients may present following disease spread which may manifest with localizing symptoms such as a lump in the axilla, bony pain, jaundice, dyspnea, or neurology. In more disseminated disease, patients may also present with non-specific constitutional symptoms such as weight loss, anorexia, and night sweats.

A number of countries have introduced national breast cancer screening programs to provide early diagnosis and improve survival rates. Typically, this involves invitation of women within an at-risk age range (usually between 40 and 70 years) to undergo screening mammography every 2–3 years. The utility of such programs is contentious and there is limited evidence to suggest an associated reduction in mortality or cost-effectiveness of a population-level screening program [6]. Screening may be associated with an increased incidence of cancer, increased intervention, and treatment, and increased morbidity associated with this. In addition, there is increased use of resources, as well the increased psychological anxiety for women who are recalled for further investigation. However, advocates argue that screening enables the earlier diagnosis of breast cancers at a stage when they are more amenable to curative treatment.

1.1.2 Diagnosis

Following presentation, patients undergo a triple assessment consisting of examination, imaging and sampling, and pathological assessment of a tissue sample [7]. Examination includes bimanual palpation of the breasts and the axilla for nodes, as well as clinical assessment for distant or systemic metastases (bone, liver, lung, and brain being common metastatic sites). Imaging consists of radiographic mammography of both breasts as well as ultrasound assessment of the breast and regional lymph nodes on the affected side. MRI is not routinely used but may be considered as an adjunct problem-solving tool depending on specific clinical indications. Tissue sampling is typically performed via core needle biopsy (or occasionally where this is not possible, fine needle aspirate (FNA) may be adequate). Suspicious lymph nodes identified by examination or imaging should also be sampled either by FNA or core biopsy. For patients undergoing operative management with curative intent, the status of the sentinel node should also be assessed for disease involvement.

1.1.3   Staging and Classification

Systemic staging may be required in locally advanced or inflammatory breast cancer, and can be done using computed tomography (CT), bone scintigraphy, and increasingly ^{18}F-FDG PET-CT. Assessment for cerebral metastases can be made with MRI.

Classification should be made according to the World Health Organization (WHO) histopathological classification and the TNM staging system (Table 1.2 and appendix). The most common histological subtypes of breast cancer are invasive ductal carcinoma, ductal carcinoma in situ, and invasive lobular carcinoma. In addition, pathology reports should include assessment of estrogen receptor (ER), progesterone receptor (PR), and human epidermal growth factor 2 receptor (HER2) status. These biomarkers have important implications in terms of prognostication and guiding therapy selection. Other markers of proliferation such as mitotic index or Ki67 labeling can provide additional prognostic information.

Table 1.2 Simplified breast cancer TNM staging [8]

Primary tumor (T)	
1	Tumor ≤20 mm in greatest dimension
2	Tumor >20 mm but ≤50 mm in greatest dimension
3	Tumor >50 mm in greatest dimension
4	Any tumor with direct extension to the chest wall or skin
Regional lymph nodes (N)	
1	Metastases in one to three axillary (level I, II) lymph nodes; or metastases in internal mammary nodes not clinically detected
2	Metastases in four to nine axillary lymph nodes (level I, II); or clinically detected metastases to internal mammary nodes
3	Metastases in ten or more axillary lymph nodes (level I, II); or clinically detected metastases to internal mammary nodes with one or more positive axillary lymph nodes (level I, II); or metastases in infraclavicular nodes (level III); or metastases to supraclavicular nodes
Distant metastases (M)	
1	No evidence of distant metastases
2	Evidence of distant metastases

Surgery remains the mainstay of curative management, and may or may not be breast conserving. Axillary clearance surgery and its associated morbidity including lymphedema can be mitigated in low-risk patients through sentinel node sampling during the primary surgery.

Radiotherapy and systemic therapies may be used in an adjuvant or a neo-adjuvant context. In advanced disease, a number of systemic therapies are available including conventional chemotherapy (including anthracycline-based regimens and paclitaxel), hormone therapy (such as tamoxifen and aromatase inhibitors), targeted therapies (such as trastuzumab/tradename Herceptin or antibody-drug conjugate derivatives such as trastuzumab emtansine/tradename Kadcyla or trastuzumab deruxtecan/tradename Enhertu) as well as a number of emerging immunotherapies.

1.1.4 Outcomes

The risk of recurrence following curative treatment is highest within 2 years, although patients have a substantial risk of recurrence for at least 20 years following diagnosis. Current follow-up protocols advise follow-up every 3–4 months for the first 2 years, every 6 months for the next 3 years, and then annually thereafter. Follow-up should include a thorough history and examination and be supplemented with annual imaging.

Ten-year survival figures for breast cancer now exceed 70% in most European countries, although this varies substantially depending on stage at presentation ranging from in excess of 90% for local disease to roughly 10% for metastatic disease [9]. Over time, breast cancer survival is improving across the developed world; a change which has largely been attributed to the development of adjuvant chemotherapy [10].

References

1. Fitzmaurice C, Allen C, Barber RM, Barregard L, Bhutta ZA, Brenner H, Dicker DJ, Chimed-Orchir O, Dandona R, Dandona L. Global, regional, and national cancer incidence, mortality, years of life lost, years lived with disability, and disability-adjusted life-years for 32 cancer groups, 1990 to 2015: a systematic analysis for the global burden of disease study. JAMA Oncol. 2017;3(4):524–48.
2. Porter PL. Global trends in breast cancer incidence and mortality. Salud pública Méx. 2009;51:s141–6.
3. American Cancer Society (2017) Breast cancer facts & figures 2017–2018. Atlanta. https://www.cancer.org/content/dam/cancer-org/research/cancer-facts-and-statistics/breast-cancer-facts-and-figures/breast-cancer-facts-and-figures-2017-2018.pdf
4. Antoniou A, Pharoah PDP, Narod S, Risch HA, Eyfjord JE, Hopper JL, Loman N, Olsson H, Johannsson O, Borg Å. Average risks of breast and ovarian cancer associated with BRCA1 or BRCA2 mutations detected in case series unselected for family history: a combined analysis of 22 studies. Am J Hum Genet. 2003;72(5):1117–30.

5. Key T, Appleby P, Barnes I, Reeves G. Endogenous sex hormones and breast cancer in postmenopausal women: reanalysis of nine prospective studies. J Natl Cancer Inst. 2002;94(8):606–16.
6. Gøtzsche PC, Jørgensen KJ. Screening for breast cancer with mammography. Cochrane Database Syst Rev. 2013;2013(6):CD001877.
7. Senkus E, Kyriakides S, Ohno S, Penault-Llorca F, Poortmans P, Rutgers E, Zackrisson S, Cardoso F. Primary breast cancer: ESMO Clinical Practice Guidelines for diagnosis, treatment and follow-up. Ann Oncol. 2015;26(suppl_5):v8–v30.
8. NCCN Clinical Practice Guidelines in Oncology: breast cancer. Version 1.2016. National Comprehensive Cancer Network
9. Allemani C, Minicozzi P, Berrino F, Bastiaannet E, Gavin A, Galceran J, Ameijide A, Siesling S, Mangone L, Ardanaz E. Predictions of survival up to 10 years after diagnosis for European women with breast cancer in 2000–2002. Int J Cancer. 2013;132(10):2404–12.
10. Narod SA, Iqbal J, Miller AB. Why have breast cancer mortality rates declined? J Cancer Policy. 2015;5:8–17.

Pathology of Breast Cancer

2

Anupama Nayak

Contents

Breast cancer is a leading cause of cancer-related mortality in women worldwide. In general, the majority of breast carcinomas are adenocarcinomas that develop from mammary epithelial cells of the terminal duct lobular unit (TDLU). Invasive carcinoma is classified into special morphologic subtypes primarily based on their distinctive histological features that are also linked to specific clinical and biological behavior.

2.1 Invasive Breast Carcinoma of No Special Type (IC-NST)

Invasive breast carcinoma (NST) is the term used for a heterogeneous group of tumors that lack sufficient characteristics to be classified as a specific histological subtype, for example, lobular, tubular, or mucinous carcinoma [1]. Approximately

A. Nayak (✉)

Department of Pathology and Laboratory Medicine, Perelman School of Medicine, Hospital of the University of Pennsylvania, Philadelphia, PA, USA
e-mail: Anupma.nayak@pennmedicine.upenn.edu

Fig. 2.1 Invasive breast carcinoma of no special type

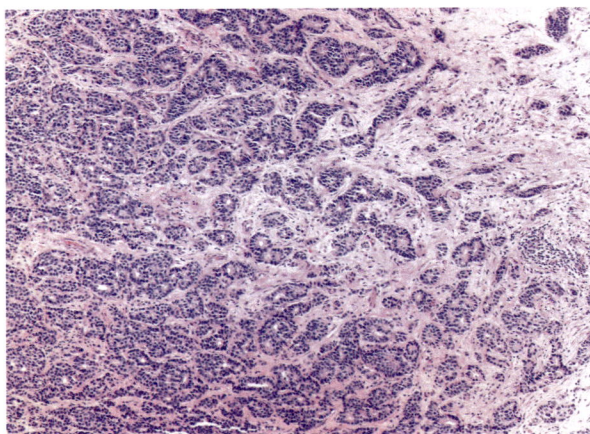

75% of invasive cancers fall into this category [2]. Architecturally, the tumor cells may be arranged in glands, cords, trabeculae, solid or syncytial growth patterns (Fig. 2.1). The tumor cells may have moderate to abundant cytoplasm with mild to severe nuclear pleomorphism. The mitotic activity may vary and necrosis may be present either focal or occasionally extensive. The tumor stroma may be cellular with desmoplastic reaction or markedly sclerotic. In a few cases, prominent lymphoplasmacytic infiltrate is identified.

2.2   Invasive Lobular Carcinoma

Invasive lobular carcinoma accounts for 5–15% of invasive breast cancers and includes many histologic variants, e.g., *classic, pleomorphic, solid, alveolar, tubulolobular*, and *mixed* [1]. Classic ILC, the most common type of ILC, is composed of non-cohesive tumor cells dispersed individually or in a single-file linear pattern within fibrous stroma (Fig. 2.2). Infiltrating tumor cells are frequently arranged in a concentric pattern around normal ducts, a feature known as *targetoid* growth pattern. Cytologically, the tumor cells exhibit low-grade nuclear atypia, and eosinophilic cytoplasm. Intracytoplasmic lumina is a characteristic feature of lobular cells, sometimes resulting in a signet ring cell appearance. Mitotic figures are rare and so are the desmoplasia and lymphoplasmacytic reactions. The *solid* variant of ILC is characterized by large sheets of uniform cells of lobular morphology with no or little intervening stroma. The cells are dyscohesive and slightly more pleomorphic and mitotically active than the classic ILC. In the *alveolar* variant, tumor cells are arranged in small nests of at least 20 cells separated by thin bands of fibrous stroma.

Fig. 2.2 Invasive lobular carcinoma

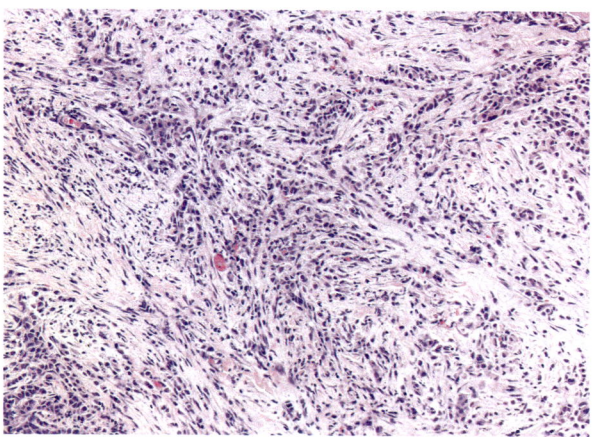

The *tubulolobular* variant is composed of a mixture of well-differentiated tubular-like glands and dyscohesive lobular cells arranged in a single-file pattern. The *pleomorphic* variant of ILC retains the distinctive growth pattern of classic ILC but exhibits a greater degree of cellular atypia and pleomorphism. The tumor cells may also show apocrine, histiocytoid, and signet cell differentiation. This variant is reported to have worse clinical behavior among all subtypes of ILC and tends to respond better to systemic chemotherapy [3, 4]. Often, the tumor shows an admixture of two or more of the above variants and therefore classified as a *mixed* variant of ILC. A vast majority of ILCs (80–100%) lose expression of membrane staining for E-cadherin/beta-catenin, a feature corroborated by molecular studies showing deletion of or truncated mutations in the E-cadherin gene. Immunohistochemically, this feature is often used to differentiate lobular carcinomas from ductal carcinomas [5].

2.3   Invasive Tubular Carcinoma

Invasive tubular carcinoma (2% of all invasive carcinomas) is a special type of breast carcinoma with a favorable prognosis than IDC, NST [1]. It is characterized by haphazard proliferation of oval, rounded, or angulated tubules with well-formed open lumens (Fig. 2.3). The tubules are lined by a single layer of epithelial cells with basally oriented nuclei having minimal nuclear atypia and scant mitotic figures. The tubules may show cytoplasmic apical snouts and are often accompanied by desmoplastic stroma or fibroelastosis. Calcifications in association with tumor glands, stroma, or associated in situ carcinoma are frequently identified.

Fig. 2.3 Invasive tubular carcinoma

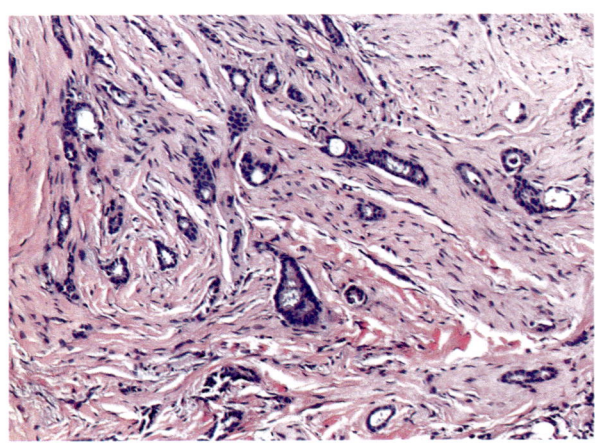

2.4   Invasive Mucinous Carcinoma

Pure mucinous carcinoma (2% of all breast carcinomas), also known as colloid carcinoma, is a special type of invasive breast carcinoma with a better prognosis than IDC, NST [1]. It is characterized by the presence of abundant extracellular mucin around the nests of tumor cells. The neoplastic cells are typically dispersed within extracellular mucin in small clusters, sheets, glandular, cribriform, papillary, or micropapillary configurations (Fig. 2.4). Pure mucinous carcinoma is diagnosed only when >90% of the tumor is mucinous [1]. Tumors containing a mixture of mucinous and non-mucinous components (>10% non-mucinous component) are distinguished from pure mucinous carcinoma as the prognoses are different. Mucinous carcinomas are usually well-differentiated with no or mild nuclear atypia and scant mitotic activity. A subgroup of mucinous carcinoma shows neuroendocrine differentiation as defined by cytoplasmic argyrophilia or immunoreactivity to neuroendocrine markers (chromogranin and synaptophysin) [6].

Fig. 2.4 Invasive
mucinous carcinoma

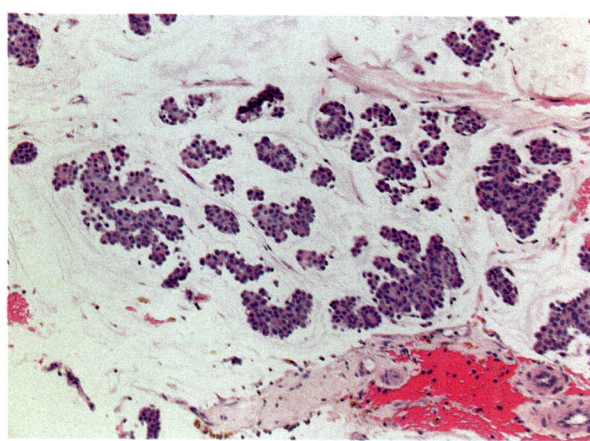

2.5   Invasive Micropapillary Carcinoma

Invasive micropapillary carcinoma (IMP) is a distinct subtype of invasive breast carcinoma with aggressive behavior when compared to IDC and NST. Pure forms of IMP are relatively rare (<2% of all invasive carcinomas) [1]. In a vast majority of cases, IMP is admixed with IC-NST. Characteristically, the tumor cells with micropapillary, morular, or tubuloalveolar patterns are suspended in clear spaces. The micropapillary clusters by definition, lack fibrovascular cores, unlike true papillary carcinoma. In the tubuloalveolar pattern, a central lumen is appreciated. The cells in micropapillary carcinoma have reversed polarity (also known as inside-out growth pattern), where the apical surface of cells is polarized to the outside (Fig. 2.5) [7]. The individual tumor cells have moderate to abundant eosinophilic cytoplasm, intermediate to high-grade nuclei, and frequent mitoses. These tumors have a high propensity for lymphatic spread, and consequent axillary lymph node and distant metastases [8]. The micropapillary architecture is interestingly retained in lymph nodes and distant metastatic sites.

Fig. 2.5 Invasive
micropapillary carcinoma

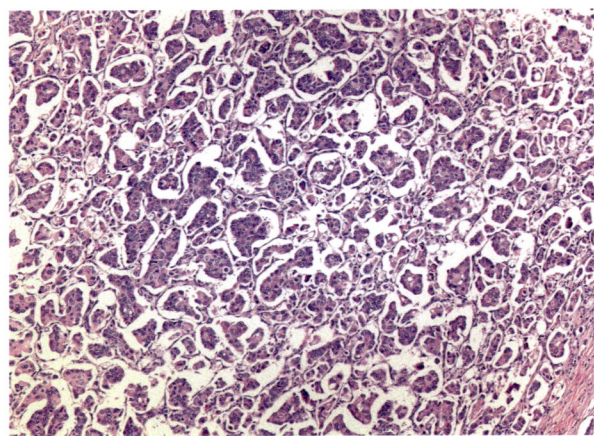

2.6   Invasive Metaplastic Carcinoma

Metaplastic carcinoma (<1% of all invasive breast carcinomas) is a heterogeneous group of invasive breast cancers displaying adenocarcinoma, squamous, spindle cell, and/or heterologous mesenchymal differentiation (chondroid, osseous, rhabdomyoid, etc.) (Fig. 2.6) [1]. The degree of metaplasia varies from rare microscopic foci in an otherwise usual invasive ductal carcinoma to complete replacement of glandular component by the metaplastic component. A vast majority of metaplastic carcinomas exhibit high-grade cytology; however, some variants such as *low-grade fibromatosis-like metaplastic carcinoma* and *low-grade adenosquamous carcinoma* may appear deceptively benign and are often misdiagnosed as fibromatosis, nodular fasciitis, reactive granulation tissue, or squamous metaplasia. Metaplastic carcinomas, in general, have a significantly lower rate of axillary nodal metastases than conventional ductal and lobular carcinomas. Recent survival studies have not found any major difference in recurrence and survival when matched with usual invasive ductal carcinomas [1].

Fig. 2.6 Invasive
metaplastic carcinoma with
squamous differentiation

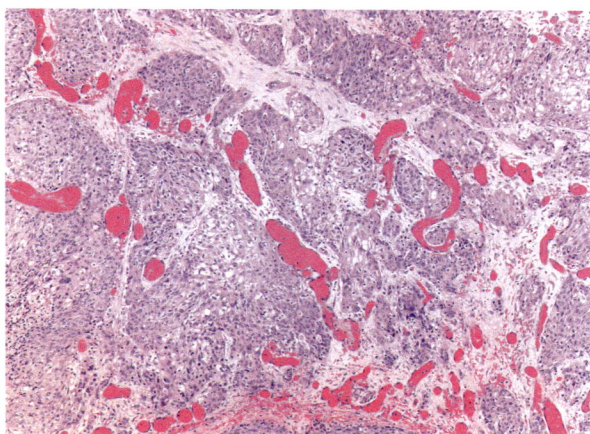

2.7   Invasive Carcinoma with Medullary Features

Invasive carcinoma with medullary features is a rare group of breast cancers representing <1% of all invasive carcinomas [1]. Morphologically, the tumor is characterized by microscopic circumscription, predominant syncytial growth pattern with indistinct cell borders of at least 75% of the tumor, associated diffuse lymphoplasmacytic infiltrate, and a lack of intraductal component or glandular differentiation. These tumors are more common in young patients with BRCA1 germline mutation and are associated with relatively better outcomes when compared with IC-NST, possibly due to associated dense lymphoplasmacytic infiltrate [1].

2.8   Adenoid Cystic Carcinoma (AdCC)

Adenoid cystic carcinoma is a rare salivary gland type tumor of breast accounting for <1% of all breast cancers [1]. The tumors are composed of a dual cell population of luminal epithelial cells and myoepithelial cells. Architecturally, they may exhibit cribriform (sieve-like), tubular, trabecular, and/or solid growth patterns. The most common pattern is cribriform with variably sized, smoothly contoured nests of small round cells perforated by small rigid punched-out spaces (lumens) like a sieve

Fig. 2.7 Adenoid cystic carcinoma

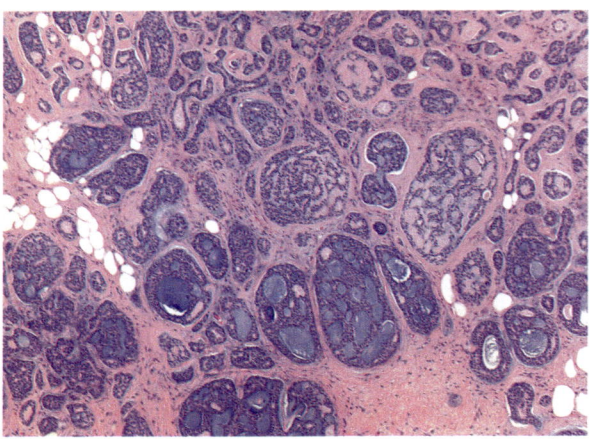

(Fig. 2.7). The spaces are of two types: pseudolumens and true glandular spaces. The pseudolumens are formed by intratumoral invagination of the stroma composed of basophilic myxoid substance or eosinophilic hyalinized collagen, and are lined by single or multiple layers of basaloid cells. The true glandular spaces are less common, contain eosinophilic granular secretions and are lined by cuboidal cells with eosinophilic cytoplasm. Sebaceous differentiation and squamous metaplasia may be seen in a few cases. Similar to salivary gland AdCCs, breast AdCCs frequently show recurrent chromosomal translocation t(6;9) resulting in fusion of the oncogene *MYB* (6q22-q23) with the transcription factor *NFIB* (9p23-p24). Interestingly, contrary to salivary gland AdCCs, breast AdCCs have indolent behavior with an extremely low incidence of axillary nodal metastases and rare case reports of distant metastases, mostly to lung [1].

2.9 Prognostic and Predictive Factors

Histologic grade—is one of the important prognostic features of invasive breast carcinomas. The tumor is graded based on the Elston-Ellis modification of the Scarff-Bloom Richardson (SBR) grading system (Nottingham Grading System) using three characteristics of the tumor: the degree of gland/tubule formation, nuclear pleomorphism, and mitotic activity [9]. Each of the three variables is scored on a scale of 1–3 and added to derive a final SBR score and Grade/Differentiation as shown in Table 2.1.

Biomarkers—All invasive breast carcinomas are assessed for estrogen receptor (ER), progesterone receptor (PR), and Human epidermal growth factor receptor 2 (HER2) status using ASCO-CAP guidelines to determine the prognosis and to predict the response to endocrine and/or anti-HER2 therapy. Approximately 70–80% of breast carcinomas are ER/PR positive. 15–20% are HER2 positive and the remaining 10–15% are triple negative [1]. The usual biomarker pattern of various subtypes of invasive cancers is shown in Table 2.2.

Table 2.1 Elston-Ellis modification of Scarff-Bloom-Richardson grading system for breast carcinoma (Nottingham Grading System)

Tubule formation				Score
>75% of tumor				1
10–75% of tumor				2
<10% of tumor				3
Nuclear pleomorphism				
Small, regular, uniform nuclei				1
Moderate increase in size and variability				2
Marked variation (>3 times)				3
Mitotic activity				
Field area (mm²)	0.152	0.274	0.312	
Mitotic count				
	0–5	0–9	0–11	1
	6–10	10–19	12–22	2
	>11	>20	>23	3

Add up the score for each variable for total score (minimum score 3 and maximum score 9): Total score: 3–5 (Grade 1; well-differentiated): 6–7 (Grade 2; moderately differentiated): 8–9 (Grade 3; poorly differentiated)

Table 2.2 Biomarker status and prognosis of major histologic subtypes of invasive breast carcinomas

Histologic type	Typical biomarkers	Prognosis
Invasive tubular carcinoma	ER+/PR+/HER2−	Favorable
Invasive mucinous carcinoma	ER+/PR+/HER2−	Favorable
Invasive carcinoma with medullary features	ER−/PR−/HER2− (triple negative)	Favorable
Invasive micropapillary carcinoma	Variable	Higher rate of lymph node and distant metastases
Adenoid cystic carcinoma	ER−/PR−/HER2− (triple negative)	Favorable
Invasive metaplastic carcinoma	ER−/PR−/HER2− (triple negative)	Lower rate of lymph node metastases, otherwise similar to matched IC-NST
Invasive lobular carcinoma	ER+/PR+/HER2− *15% of Pleomorphic ILC may be HER2+	Variable
Invasive carcinoma, NST	Variable	Variable

Histologic subtype (discussed above), axillary lymph node status (most important prognostic factor), tumor size, margin status, and *lymphovascular invasion* are other prognostic factors that are mandatory to be evaluated and reported in a pathology report [1].

References

1. WHO Classification of Tumours of the Breast. IARC WHO classification of tumours. Geneva: World Health Organization; 2012.
2. Li CI, Daling JR, Malone KE, et al. Relationship between established breast cancer risk factors and risk of seven different histologic types of invasive breast cancer. Cancer Epidemiol Biomark Prev. 2006;15:946–54.
3. Middleton LP, Palacios DM, Bryant BR, Krebs P, Otis CN, Merino MJ. Pleomorphic lobular carcinoma: morphology, immunohistochemistry, and molecular analysis. Am J Surg Pathol. 2000;24:1650–6.
4. Katz A, Saad ED, Porter P, Pusztai L. Primary systemic chemotherapy of invasive lobular carcinoma of the breast. Lancet Oncol. 2007;8:55–62.
5. Moll R, Mitze M, Frixen UH, Birchmeier W. Differential loss of E-cadherin expression in infiltrating ductal and lobular breast carcinomas. Am J Pathol. 1993;143:1731–42.
6. Scopsi L, Andreola S, Pilotti S, et al. Mucinous carcinoma of the breast. A clinicopathologic, histochemical, and immunocytochemical study with special reference to neuroendocrine differentiation. Am J Surg Pathol. 1994;18:702–11.
7. Siriaunkgul S, Tavassoli FA. Invasive micropapillary carcinoma of the breast. Mod Pathol. 1993;6:660–2.
8. Zekioglu O, Erhan Y, Ciris M, Bayramoglu H, Ozdemir N. Invasive micropapillary carcinoma of the breast: high incidence of lymph node metastasis with extranodal extension and its immunohistochemical profile compared with invasive ductal carcinoma. Histopathology. 2004;44:18–23.
9. Elston CW, Ellis IO. Pathological prognostic factors in breast cancer I. The value of histological grade in breast cancer: experience from a large study with long-term follow-up. Histopathology. 1991;19:403–10.

Management of Breast Cancer

3

Panagiotis Koliou and Rob Stein

Contents

The goals of breast cancer treatment are determined by the extent of disease. Early breast cancer, which is a disease confined to the breast and regional lymph nodes, is treated with curative intent using a multimodality approach. Local disease eradication is achieved by surgery, with or without radiotherapy. Systemic treatments with

P. Koliou
Royal Surrey NHS Foundation Trust, Guildford, UK

University College London Hospitals NHS Foundation trust, London, UK
e-mail: panagiotis.koliou@nhs.net

R. Stein (✉)
Royal Surrey NHS Foundation Trust, Guildford, UK
e-mail: r.stein@ucl.ac.uk

anti-oestrogens, cytotoxic chemotherapy, and targeted agents such as anti-HER2 therapy are given to eradicate undetectable micro-metastases; the choice of modalities is dictated by the characteristics of the tumour. Advanced or metastatic breast cancer (stage IV disease) on the contrary is incurable so the goals of treatment are to relieve symptoms and prolong life. Because of the disseminated nature of the disease, the primary treatment modality is systemic, the exact modality being determined by tumour biology as in early disease. Surgery has little role to play in the management of advanced disease but radiotherapy is widely used to provide valuable palliation for local symptoms such as bone pain. Imaging plays an essential role at all stages of treatment in defining the extent of disease to aid treatment planning and in monitoring treatment response with PET-CT becoming an increasingly important tool.

3.1 Local Management of Early Breast Cancer

3.1.1 Pure Non-Invasive Carcinoma: Ductal Carcinoma In Situ

Ductal Carcinoma in Situ (DCIS) continues to be a subject of controversy in breast cancer because whilst many such lesions progress to invasive disease, a significant proportion does not. In the absence of a reliable method of identifying DCIS with low risk of progression, the normal management is excision. Postoperative radiotherapy and anti-oestrogen treatment for oestrogen receptor-positive (ER-positive) DCIS may be used to reduce the risk of local recurrence, which in 50% of cases will be invasive. It is standard practice to perform annual surveillance mammography for 5 years following treatment.

3.1.2 Lobular Carcinoma In Situ (LCIS) or Lobular Neoplasia

Pure LCIS is no longer considered to be a pre-malignant entity as progression to invasive disease is rare, but is rather a risk factor for the future development of invasive disease. Controversy exists regarding whether surgical excision LCIS diagnosed by core biopsy that is not associated with a structural mammographic abnormality or residual calcifications should be performed. There is evidence that the pleomorphic variant of LCIS does have the potential to progress and should be treated like higher risk DCIS. Women with LCIS may be offered anti-oestrogen treatment to reduce the risk of subsequent development of invasive disease. Annual surveillance mammography is recommended.

3.1.3 Early-stage Invasive Breast Cancer

(usually considered as stage I, IIA [T1–2 N0] and a subset of stage IIB disease [T2N1]).

Patients with early-stage breast cancer undergo primary surgery (local excision/lumpectomy or mastectomy) together with axillary surgery, generally dual-tracer sentinel lymph node biopsy in the absence of proven axillary involvement. Radiation therapy (RT) to the breast is considered to be the standard of care following local excision because of the otherwise high rate of local recurrence. Post-mastectomy RT to the chest wall may be beneficial in those cases where 1–3 axillary lymph nodes are involved (stage IIB disease) and is standard when there are 4 or more involved nodes.

The vast majority of these patients have no evidence of metastatic disease at diagnosis, but because of the risk of metastatic relapse, are ordinarily advised preventative (adjuvant) systemic therapy. The approach to adjuvant treatment depends on predicted drug sensitivity and on risk, both of which are influenced by tumour characteristics including grade combined with TNM stage at presentation. Systemic treatment is further discussed below. Clinical guidance on anatomic staging is provided by the American Joint Committee on Cancer (AJCC) Staging Manual, currently the eighth edition.

3.1.4 Locally Advanced Breast Cancer

(includes a subset of patients with stage IIB disease [T3N0] and patients with stage IIIA to IIIC disease).

This group of patients is at high risk of relapse. Overt metastases are present at diagnosis in a significant proportion so initial assessment should involve whole-body imaging; cranial imaging is infrequently undertaken in the absence of symptoms. Conventional staging is with contrast-enhanced CT of the chest, abdomen, and pelvis usually combined with a radionuclide bone scan as supported by international guidelines [1]. PET-CT imaging may be undertaken to clarify the nature of indeterminate lesions seen on diagnostic scans although there is a move toward PET-CT as a substitute for conventional diagnostic imaging as the technology becomes more readily available.

Management is with multimodality therapy as with earlier-stage disease but there is a greater emphasis on systemic treatment. In many cases, patients with locally advanced breast cancer are treated with neoadjuvant systemic therapy, usually chemotherapy. The goal of treatment is to induce a tumour response before surgery to facilitate breast conservation. Imaging with either MRI or ultrasound is used to monitor response. In historic clinical trials, the long-term outcome from neoadjuvant therapy is the same as for initial surgery followed by adjuvant treatment [2]. There is however some evidence that patients with biologically high-risk breast cancer subtypes are disadvantaged by delay in the initiation of systemic therapy and it is therefore becoming common to treat with chemotherapy and where appropriate, anti-HER2 therapy in the neoadjuvant setting. Currently, all patients should undergo surgery following neoadjuvant systemic therapy, even where there is a complete clinical and/or radiological response. This approach is being questioned and is the subject of ongoing trials. Those patients who experience progression during neoadjuvant treatment should proceed with surgery where possible, rather than switching treatment regimens.

3.1.5   T4 and Inflammatory Breast Cancer

T4 tumours are locally advanced cancers where the tumour involves either the chest wall, overlying skin, or both. Inflammatory breast cancer (IBC) forms a rare subset of T4 tumours accounting for 0.5–2% of invasive breast cancers. Patients typically present with a short (typically a few weeks) history of breast pain or a rapidly growing, self-diagnosed breast lump [3]. On presentation, almost all women with IBC have lymph node involvement, and approximately one-third will additionally have overt distant metastases [4, 5]. IBC is associated with a higher prevalence of visceral metastases compared with other forms of breast cancer due to early and aggressive hematogenous spread. The diagnosis of IBC is clinical as there are no pathognomonic defining features although involvement of the overlying skin is common. A significant proportion of IBC cases are HER2 positive.

Management of T4 disease is as for locally advanced disease. However, as T4 tumours are considered to be inoperable, neoadjuvant treatment to downstage the tumour and bring it under control is the norm. Surgery is usually a mastectomy. The great majority of patients will undergo post-surgical radiotherapy ordinarily including the supraclavicular region to prevent nodal recurrence. Radiotherapy fields, particularly for these more advanced tumours are increasingly being extended to the internal mammary node chain even in the absence of imaging evidence for disease as sub-clinical involvement is common.

3.2   Breast Cancer Subtypes and Systemic Therapy

Systemic therapy refers to the medical treatment of breast cancer using endocrine therapy, chemotherapy, and biologic therapy. The approach to systemic therapy is driven by tumour biology as tumour characteristics predict which patients are likely to benefit from specific types of therapy. The pioneering work of Perou and collaborators identified the "intrinsic subtypes" of breast cancer which are defined by gene expression patterns and which have very different natural histories. The intrinsic subtypes were initially described using microarray technology [6] and more recently using the PAM50 50-gene signature [7]. PAM50 subtyping is now available commercially but is not in widespread use. The PAM50 subtypes are approximately recapitulated by patterns of receptor expression and proliferation markers such as Ki67 (Table 3.1). Of note, luminal A breast cancer, which is the most frequent subtype diagnosed in the developed world, has a good prognosis whilst other subtypes are much more likely to recur and are consequently treated more aggressively.

Response to and hence benefit from treatment is predicted by receptor expression and additionally by PAM50 subtype. For example, patients with oestrogen receptor-positive (ER-positive) tumours are likely to benefit from endocrine therapy whilst ER-negative disease is resistant to this treatment modality. The progesterone receptor (PR) is best thought of as a prognostic marker; ER-negative PR-positive tumours are rare. Patients with human epidermal growth factor receptor 2 (HER2)-positive cancers usually benefit from treatment using HER2-directed treatment such as the monoclonal antibody, trastuzumab or in combination with pertuzumab. There are no

Table 3.1 Surrogates for breast cancer molecular subtypes after the St. Gallen consensus 2013 [8]

	ER	PR	HER2	Ki-67
Luminal A[a]	+	+	−	Low (<14%)
Luminal B (HER2-)[b]	+	−/low	−	High (≥14%)
Luminal B (HER2+)	+	Any	Amplified	Any
HER2-enriched	−	−	Amplified	N/A
Triple-negative/basal-like	−	−	−	N/A

ER, oestrogen receptor; PR, progesterone receptor; HER2, human epidermal growth factor receptor 2; N/A, not applicable.
[a]A PR cut-point of ≥20% expression best corresponds to luminal A subtype when distinguishing between luminal A-like and luminal B-like tumours
[b]ER-positive and HER2-negative and at least one of: Ki-67 high, PR-negative, or low, or recurrence risk high

tests that convincingly predict chemotherapy sensitivity, particularly for ER-positive HER2-negative tumours. Although claims have been made that some multi-gene pathology tests such as Oncotype DX®, also known as the 21-gene recurrence score have this property [9, 10], this remains controversial [11].

There is incontrovertible evidence that overall, chemotherapy reduces the risk of breast cancer recurrence and death by about one-third [12]. Chemotherapy is routinely offered to all patients with triple-negative and or HER2-positive disease (in which case it is combined with HER2-targeted therapy) except in very early disease (particularly tumour size <5 mm with no nodal spread) where the individual risk of recurrence is too low to justify the likely toxicity. Patients with these tumour types are frequently treated in the neoadjuvant setting, especially those with tumours above 2 cm in size or with node positive disease. Chemotherapy for patients with early-stage HER2-negative luminal-type tumours, particularly luminal A, is more controversial. It is frequently advised for those whose tumours have high-risk characteristics, such as high-grade, large size (≥2 cm), pathologically involved lymph nodes, high proliferation indices where measured, and "high risk" biology defined by Oncotype DX and related gene expression tests. For other patients, we prefer not to administer chemotherapy because of the likely poor risk-benefit ratio. Multi-gene pathology tests have convincingly demonstrated their superiority over conventional grade in the identification of these patients with low recurrence risk who can safely avoid chemotherapy [11] and are widely used for this purpose. Where chemotherapy is indicated, the most commonly used treatment regimens are administered 3-weekly for between 4 and 8 cycles depending on perceived risk and usually contain alkylating agents (cyclophosphamide), an anthracycline and a taxane.

Neoadjuvant treatment for patients with HER2-positive tumours normally consists of dual HER2-targeted therapy with trastuzumab and pertuzumab combined with chemotherapy, which has extraordinarily high response rates. Where this approach achieves a pathological complete response at surgery, the current standard of care is for the continuation of trastuzumab as monotherapy (combined with anti-oestrogens where appropriate) to give a total of 12 months of treatment. The antibody-drug conjugate, trustuzumab emtansine (T-DM1) is a superior option to adjuvant trastuzumab where residual disease is found in the breast or nodes at surgery [13].

Endocrine therapy is probably the most important component of systemic treatment for luminal breast cancers and clearly reduces the risk of recurrence and death. The selection of endocrine therapy is made according to menopausal status. The advised minimum duration of adjuvant treatment is 5 years with evidence of additional benefit for up to 10 years for those with adverse features such as more advanced stage or luminal B-like features. Endocrine therapy has additionally been shown to reduce the risk of developing contralateral tumours. Neoadjuvant endocrine treatment used to downstage locally advanced luminal A-type disease is more likely to succeed than chemotherapy.

3.3   Patient Follow-Up

Cancer survivors who have completed treatment for breast cancer undergo regular surveillance. Annual mammography should be performed, typically for 5 years. The routine use of breast magnetic resonance imaging (MRI) or whole-breast ultrasound is not recommended for breast cancer survivors although MRI has a place for the young with mammographically dense breasts. Laboratory tests and whole-body imaging in asymptomatic patients is not recommended.

3.4   Male Breast Cancer

This is a rare condition accounting for 0.7% of diagnoses in the UK. It is particularly infrequent under the age of 50 years. Male breast cancer is overwhelmingly ER-positive and although biological differences from the common female ER-positive disease are increasingly recognised, there is no fundamental difference between the two. The principles of management are therefore the same although there are some differences in detail.

3.5   Stage IV or Metastatic Breast Cancer

The majority of patients who develop metastatic breast cancer, which is probably 20–25% of patients presenting with invasive primary disease, experience distant recurrence at a variable interval following treatment for early disease [14]. Around 6–7% of patients have stage IV disease when newly diagnosed. UK statistics show that for this latter group, only 15% remain alive at 5 years [14]. Survival estimates for those who experience metastatic relapse are consistent although the data are inherently more difficult to collect.

As metastatic breast is considered to be an incurable condition, the aim of treatment is disease control rather than eradication. Systemic therapy is the primary treatment modality with local treatments such as radiotherapy and occasionally surgery being reserved for relief of troublesome symptoms such as bone pain. The characteristics of the disease and hence the basic approach to systemic therapy usually resemble those of the primary tumour. Bone is the single most common metastatic site and is frequently the only site for luminal A tumours. Visceral metastases tend to dominate non-luminal disease.

Up to 15% of tumours have discordant ER and HER2 status compared with the primary cancer, likely caused by undetected tumour heterogeneity. Therefore biopsy of a metastatic lesion in patients to confirm ER and HER2 status at first metastatic relapse is strongly recommended [15]. Measurement of PR status is not contributory. Analysis of circulating tumour cell DNA (ctDNA), sometimes called liquid biopsy, has the potential to identify therapeutically important changes in tumours. For instance, 25–40% of patients with metastatic ER-positive breast cancer have ER gene mutations, frequently polyclonal, identifiable from ctDNA analysis [16]. Such changes, which are infrequently detected in primary breast cancers may predict response or resistance to particular treatments.

Metastatic breast cancer frequently follows a relapsing and remitting pattern with the disease being brought back under control by a change of systemic treatment at relapse even within a single modality, such as change of endocrine agents. However, with time individual tumours develop increasing resistance to treatment with for instance the progression to oestrogen independence. These changes are manifest in shorter periods of disease control with individual therapeutics and a steadily rising disease burden with associated loss of quality of life.

The extent of metastatic disease and patient symptoms are important considerations when determining whether active treatment is beneficial to the patient particularly as many drugs cause significant toxicity and require frequent hospital attendance.

3.5.1 Endocrine Therapy for Metastatic Disease

Patients with ER-positive metastatic breast cancer often respond to endocrine therapy (ET), which can reduce tumour burden and consequently symptoms, with generally less toxicity than chemotherapy. Endocrine therapy is therefore the preferred treatment modality for this group of patients, particularly when bone is the dominant site of disease. The introduction of targeted agents such as PI3-kinase inhibitors and particularly cyclin-dependent kinase (CDK 4/6) inhibitors in combination with anti-oestrogens is a notable therapeutic advance [17]. CDK 4/6 inhibitors are now approved as a component of adjuvant therapy for patients with higher-risk disease [18].

As ET often works slowly, there are situations where chemotherapy, which usually achieves a more rapid response, is preferred. Some of these are described below:

End-organ dysfunction can be defined by symptoms, such as dyspnea, evidence of pulmonary lymphangitis, or abnormal liver function. The presence of visceral metastasis alone, in the absence of these findings, is not an indication to proceed with chemotherapy in lieu of a trial of ET.

Visceral crisis is defined as severe organ dysfunction as assessed by signs and symptoms, laboratory studies, and rapid progression of disease. Visceral crisis implies important organ compromise and is a clinical indication for chemotherapy, particularly since alternative treatments in the event of failure will probably not be possible.

Primary endocrine resistance is usually defined as relapse during the first 2 years of adjuvant endocrine treatment, or disease progression during the first 6 months of first line ET for metastatic breast cancer. Chemotherapy is usually the preferred next treatment.

Secondary (acquired) resistance endocrine resistance is defined as relapse during adjuvant ET but after the first 2 years, relapse within 12 months of completing adjuvant ET, or failure to achieve disease control for at least 6 months in the metastatic setting.

For patients who have initiated chemotherapy, if a satisfactory response is achieved after several cycles (3–6 months) with reduction of symptoms, it is reasonable to discontinue chemotherapy and introduce some form of endocrine treatment provided there is no evidence of endocrine independence. For others, either continuing chemotherapy (if there is evidence of response or disease stabilization), switching to another chemotherapy regimen, or shifting to palliative care only are appropriate options.

Figure 3.1 outlines the principles of treatment in newly diagnosed ER-positive, HER2-negative disease.

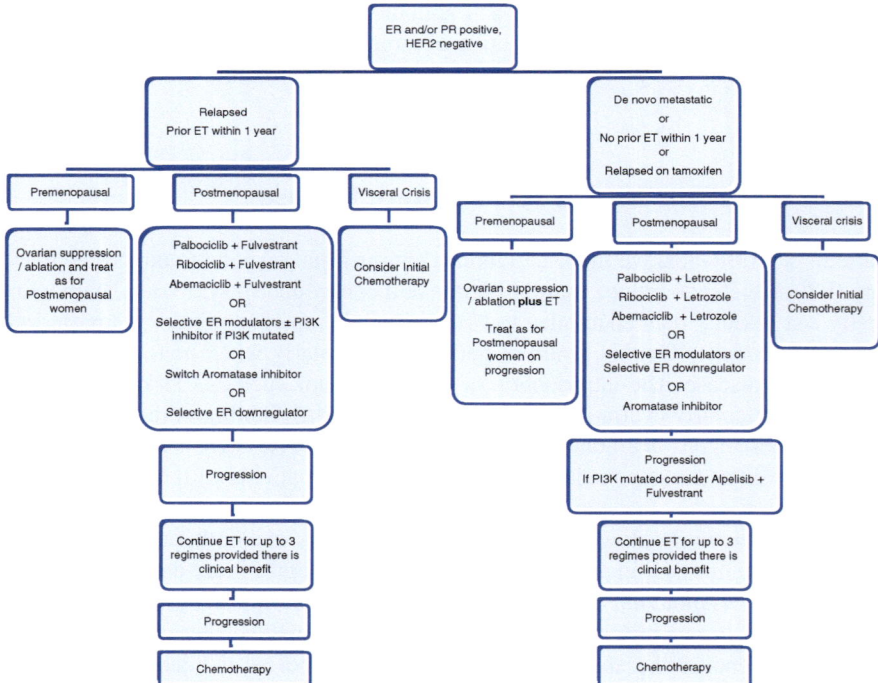

Drug names ending with "ciclib" are CDK 4/6 inhibitors. Drug names ending with "lisib" are PI3-kinase inhibitors. Selective ER modulators include tamoxifen. Selective ER downregulators or degraders include fulvestrant.

Fig. 3.1 Systemic Treatment of recurrent or stage IV disease: ER (and/or PR positive) and HER2 negative

3.5.2 HER2-Targeted Therapy for Metastatic Breast Cancer

Approximately 20% of metastatic breast cancers overexpress the HER2 receptor. In the past HER2 positive primary disease had an increased risk of local and distant recurrence with an overall worse prognosis. HER2-targeted therapy, particularly trastuzumab, however, has altered the natural course of HER2-positive breast cancer when used both as first and later line treatment [19, 20]. The introduction of dual monoclonal antibody HER2-targeted therapy with trastuzumab and pertuzumab has substantially improved outcomes for both metastatic [21] and primary disease [22].

More recently, antibody-drug conjugates (ADCs), where a targeting agent (here trastuzumab) is modified to carry a potent cytotoxic agent, have further expanded treatment options. By delivering a cytotoxic agent directly to tumour cells, ADCs have obvious advantages in terms of toxicity over conventional chemotherapy. Ado-trastuzumab emtansine (T-DM1) is now used to treat both metastatic and primary disease. Trastuzumab deruxtecan (T-DXd) has shown both non-cross-resistance to and superiority over T-DM1 at the cost of somewhat increased toxicity [23]. More importantly, it has activity against tumours that express HER2 at physiological levels without gene amplification and accordingly is licenced for the treatment of "HER2-low" metastatic breast cancer [24], thereby expanding HER2-targeted therapy to other disease subtypes. The clinical implications of this have only just begun to be explored. A further approach to treatment involves small molecule inhibitors of HER2-kinase such as lapatinib, neratinib and most recently, tucatinib. This approach has had less spectacular success than antibody-based treatments but nevertheless has clinically useful activity.

The mainstay of treatment for HER2 positive metastatic breast cancer is anti-HER2 therapy, either in the form of trastuzumab and pertuzumab combined with chemotherapy, ADCs or small molecule kinase inhibitors, currently tucatinib combined with the oral cytotoxic, capecitabine. The choice of treatment depends on prior treatment history and drug availability/ reimbursement. Following failure of initial therapy, the common practice is to continue HER2-targeted treatment. Evidence predating the current wide variety of HER2-targeted agents shows that continuation of trastuzumab in combination with cytotoxics is superior to the same cytotoxic agent given without trastuzumab [25]. Treatment choices post progression are made on the same basis as at initial metastatic relapse including of course, patient preferences. Anti-HER2 treatment in combination with endocrine therapy is an option for those with dual ER-positive HER2-positive tumours, especially if the disease is not rapidly progressive or symptomatic or is not characterized by significant visceral involvement with organ dysfunction.

CNS metastases are a particular problem for those with HER2-positive metastatic disease, possibly because of limited penetration of anti-HER2 agents across the blood–brain barrier especially during primary treatment. Treatment options include neurosurgical approaches, targeted radiotherapy, whole-brain radiotherapy, and blood–brain barrier penetrating systemic agents (Fig. 3.2).

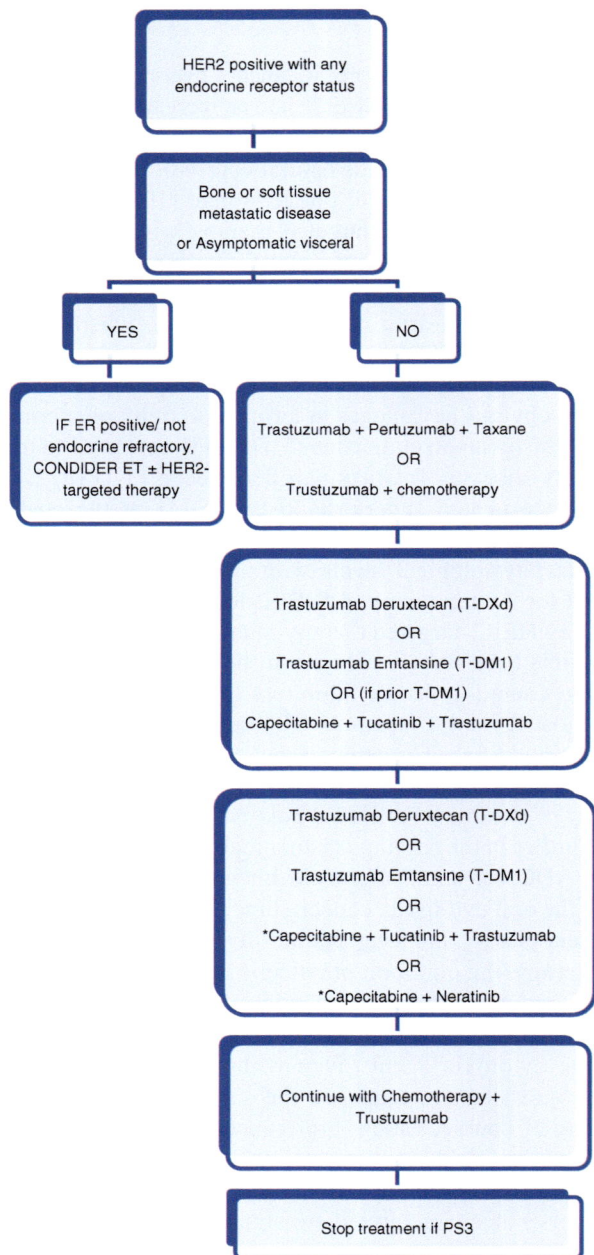

Fig. 3.2 Systemic treatment of HER2-positive disease with any hormone receptor status

3.5.3 Triple-Negative Disease

Triple-negative breast cancer (TNBC, Table 3.1) is a term that denotes cancers that have a low or absent expression of ER, PR, and HER2. TNBC accounts for approximately 15–20% of breast cancers diagnosed worldwide [14] and is more frequent in the young and in some racial groups such as women of African descent [21, 26]. TNBC is a heterogeneous entity that tends to behave more aggressively than other varieties of breast cancer [7]. The historical approach to treatment in the absence of other options has been limited to chemotherapy. Life-threatening visceral metastases, CNS involvement, and a reduced incidence of loco-regional recurrence are all features of advanced disease. [27–29] In contrast to HER2-positive disease, survival following diagnosis of CNS metastases is typically less than 6 months [30].

The choice of chemotherapy for TNBC is similar to that for ER-positive HER2-negative disease. The sequential use of single agents rather than combination therapy is preferred because of reduced toxicity and theoretically delayed development of drug resistance. Drug doses and schedules are selected to optimize the balance between efficacy and toxicity allowing treatment until progression although cumulative neurotoxicity is a problem with some drugs, particularly taxanes.

Treatment with immune checkpoint inhibitors, ordinarily in combination with chemotherapy is showing considerable promise and has led to approvals for the treatment of advanced TNBC and more recently for neoadjuvant treatment of locally advanced early disease [31]. Although a minority benefit from this approach, it is an area of intense research interest and future improvements seem highly likely. A further approach that is showing promise is the use of the ADC, sacituzumab govetican, directed against the Trop-2 antigen, which is widely expressed on the surface of solid tumours. Sacituzumab govetican is currently available as a 2nd-line treatment for metastatic TNBC [32] and has additionally been demonstrated to have activity in ER-positive disease. Although TNBC with its high rate of metastatic relapse and limited treatment options is arguably still the greatest challenge in breast cancer management today, these therapeutic developments do indicate that improvements in the outlook for these patients is on the horizon.

3.5.4 BRCA Mutant Breast Cancer

In the order of 5% of breast cancer diagnoses in women of European descent are associated with the presence of a germ-line mutation in one of the high-penetrance predisposition genes, particularly BRCA1 and BRCA2. The commonest disease phenotype associated with BRCA1 mutation is the triple-negative/basal-like sub-type whilst cancers that arise in those with BRCA2 mutations are typically ER positive [33]. The complexity of genetic testing, particularly next generation sequencing based panel testing lies outside the scope of this chapter but as the cost has fallen it is becoming increasingly frequent to offer testing to all women with younger age onset disease, particularly TNBC, regardless of family history. The presence of a BRCA mutation in women with primary disease is not associated with an adverse outcome once adjustment is made for other disease characteristics [33], and does offer additional therapeutic options at all disease stages.

The physiological role of the BRCA proteins *includes* the repair of double-strand DNA breaks. *BRCA mutation*-associated breast cancer has been shown to be particularly sensitive to certain DNA-damaging agents such as platinum agents (carboplatin or cisplatin). In particular, carboplatin has been shown to be superior to docetaxel in this population when given as first-line treatment in a randomized comparison [34, 35]. Inhibition of the enzyme polyadenosine diphosphate-ribose polymerase (PARP) exploits the DNA repair deficiency in BRCA mutant breast cancer through a process known as synthetic lethality. Several oral PARP inhibitors have been developed of which olaparib has been licenced for use in both advanced and early breast cancer on the basis of the OlympiAD and OlympiA studies [34, 36].

3.6 Assessing Treatment Response in Metastatic Breast Cancer

Assessment of treatment response and failure is a crucial component of metastatic cancer management. Clinical evaluation of patients and monitoring of blood parameters such as blood counts and serum chemistry play an important role. For instance, clinical features suggestive of progression include declining performance status; increasing pain or dyspnea; unexplained weight loss; new findings on clinical examination; increasing serum liver enzymes or bilirubin; and hypercalcemia. Conversely improvement suggests a response.

Periodic imaging studies form the cornerstone of response evaluation. In general, the same method of assessment should be used over time. Clinical trials of new agents ordinarily rely on RECIST v1.1 assessment of response typically using diagnostic CT (supplemented by isotope bone scans) performed at regular intervals such as every 8 weeks [37]. Real-world disease assessment is much more variable (Table 3.2). Intervals between scheduled imaging studies depend on the pace of disease. Therefore, imaging studies will ordinarily be performed less frequently for metastatic ER-positive disease controlled by endocrine therapy than for TNBC treated with chemotherapy.

Table 3.2 Imaging assessment of patients with metastatic breast cancer

	Assessment at baseline/disease progression	Monitoring chemotherapy response	Monitoring endocrine therapy
CT Chest/abdominal/pelvis with contrast	Yes	Every 2–4 cycles	Every 3–6 months
CT/MRI brain[a]	As required	As required	As required
Isotope bone scan	Yes	Limited value[b]	Limited value[b]
MRI (localized—e.g., bone/liver)[c]	As required	As required	As required
FDG PET-CT/MRI[d]	Potential alternative to CT	Optional	Optional

[a]CNS imaging is usually undertaken in the presence of symptoms and may be used to monitor the response of brain metastases to systemic therapy. Routine surveillance CNS imaging for TNBC and HER2-positive disease is rarely undertaken but there is a case for doing this

[b]Isotope bone scan has limited utility in monitoring treatment response because of issues such as flare

[c]MRI is widely used to assess spinal disease and in case of suspected spinal cord compression. MRI may additionally be used to monitor response in bone and where pseudo-cirrhosis is present, in liver

[d]FDG PET imaging is a potential alternative to diagnostic CT, particularly where bone metastases are a major disease component

References

1. Cardoso F, Kyriakides S, Ohno S, et al. Early breast cancer: ESMO Clinical Practice Guidelines for diagnosis, treatment and follow-up. Ann Oncol. 2019;30(8):1194–1220.
2. Early Breast Cancer Trialists' Collaborative Group (EBCTCG). Long-term outcomes for neo-adjuvant versus adjuvant chemotherapy in early breast cancer: meta-analysis of individual patient data from ten randomised trials. Lancet Oncol. 2018;19(1):27–39.
3. Matro JM, Li T, Cristofanilli M, et al. Inflammatory breast cancer management in the National Comprehensive Cancer Network: the disease, recurrence pattern, and outcome. Clin Breast Cancer. 2015;15(1):1–7.
4. Smoot RL, Koch CA, Degnim AC, et al. A single-center experience with inflammatory breast cancer, 1985–2003. Arch Surg. 2006;141(6):563–7.
5. Dawood S, Merajver SD, Viens P, et al. International expert panel on inflammatory breast cancer: consensus statement for standardized diagnosis and treatment. Ann Oncol. 2011;22(3):515–23.
6. Perou CM, Sørile T, Eisen MB, et al. Molecular portraits of human breast tumours. Nature. 2000;406(6797):747–52.
7. Parker J, Mullins M, Cheang M, et al. Supervised risk predictor of breast cancer based on intrinsic subtypes. J Clin Oncol. 2009;27(8):1160–7.

8. Goldhirsch A, Winer EP, Coates AS, et al. Personalizing the treatment of women with early breast cancer: highlights of the St Gallen international expert consensus on the primary therapy of early breast cancer 2013. Ann Oncol. 2013;24(9):2206–23.

9. Paik S, Tang G, Shak S, et al. Gene expression and benefit of chemotherapy in women with node-negative, estrogen receptor-positive breast cancer. J Clin Oncol. 2006;24(23):3726–34.

10. Albain KS, Barlow WE, Shak S, et al. Prognostic and predictive value of the 21-gene recurrence score assay in postmenopausal women with node-positive, oestrogen-receptor-positive breast cancer on chemotherapy: a retrospective analysis of a randomised trial. Lancet Oncol. 2010;11(1):55–65.

11. Ward S, Scope A, Rafia R, et al. Gene expression profiling and expanded immunohistochemistry tests to guide the use of adjuvant chemotherapy in breast cancer management: a systematic review and cost-effectiveness analysis. Health Technol Assess. 2013;17:1–302.

12. Early Breast Cancer Trialists' Collaborative Group, Peto R, Davies C, et al. Comparisons between different polychemotherapy regimens for early breast cancer: meta-analyses of long-term outcome among 100,000 women in 123 randomised trials. Lancet. 2012;379(9814):432–44.

13. von Minckwitz G, Huang CS, Mano MS, et al. Trastuzumab Emtansine for Residual Invasive HER2-Positive Breast Cancer. N Engl J Med. 2019;380:617−28.

14. Cancer Research UK. Breast Cancer Statistics. Breast Cancer Statistics [Internet]. 2023 [cited 2023 Apr 26]. Available from: https://www.cancerresearchuk.org/health-professional/cancer-statistics/statistics-by-cancer-type/breast-cancer.

15. Lindström LS, Karlsson E, Wilking UM, et al. Clinically used breast cancer markers such as estrogen receptor, progesterone receptor, and human epidermal growth factor receptor 2 are unstable throughout tumor progression. J Clin Oncol. 2012;30(21):2601–8.

16. Fribbens C, O'Leary B, Kilburn L, et al. Plasma *ESR1* mutations and the treatment of estrogen receptor–positive advanced breast cancer. J Clin Oncol. 2016;34(25):2961–8.

17. de Groot AF, Kuijpers CJ, Kroep JR. CDK4/6 inhibition in early and metastatic breast cancer: a review. Cancer Treat Rev. 2017;60:130–8.

18. Harbeck N, Rastogi P, Martin M, et al. Adjuvant abemaciclib combined with endocrine therapy for high-risk early breast cancer: updated efficacy and Ki-67 analysis from the monarchE study. Ann Oncol. 2021;32:1571−81.

19. Balduzzi S, Mantarro S, Guarneri V, et al. Trastuzumab-containing regimens for metastatic breast cancer. Cochrane Database Syst Rev. 2014;6:CD006242.

20. Swain SM, Baselga J, Kim S-B, et al. Pertuzumab, trastuzumab, and docetaxel in HER2-positive metastatic breast cancer. N Engl J Med. 2015;372(8):724–34.

21. Millikan RC, Newman B, Tse C-K, et al. Epidemiology of basal-like breast cancer. Breast Cancer Res Treat. 2008;109(1):123–39.

22. Piccart M, Procter M, Fumagalli D, et al. Adjuvant Pertuzumab and Trastuzumab in Early HER2-Positive Breast Cancer in the APHINITY Trial: 6 Years' Follow-Up. J Clin Oncol. 2021;39:1448–57.

23. Hurvitz SA, Hegg R, Chung WP, et al. Trastuzumab deruxtecan versus trastuzumab emtansine in patients with HER2-positive metastatic breast cancer: updated results from DESTINY-Breast03, a randomised, open-label, phase 3 trial. Lancet. 2023;401:105–17.

24. Modi S, Jacot W, Yamashita T, et al. Trastuzumab Deruxtecan in Previously Treated HER2-Low Advanced Breast Cancer. N Engl J Med. 2022;387:9–20.

25. Von Minckwitz G, Du Bois A, Schmidt M, et al. Trastuzumab beyond progression in human epidermal growth factor receptor 2-positive advanced breast cancer: a German Breast Group 26/Breast International Group 03-05 study. J Clin Oncol. 2009;27(12):1999–2006.

26. Parise CA, Bauer KR, Brown MM, Caggiano V. Breast cancer subtypes as defined by the estrogen receptor (ER), progesterone receptor (PR), and the human epidermal growth factor receptor 2 (HER2) among women with invasive breast cancer in California, 1999–2004. Breast J. 2009;15(6):593–602.

27. Lin NU, Vanderplas A, Hughes ME, et al. Clinicopathologic features, patterns of recurrence, and survival among women with triple-negative breast cancer in the National Comprehensive Cancer Network. Cancer. 2012;118(22):5463–72.

28. Smid M, Wang Y, Zhang Y, et al. Subtypes of breast cancer show preferential site of relapse. Cancer Res. 2008;68(9):3108–14.
29. Lin NU, Claus E, Sohl J, Razzak AR, Arnaout A, Winer EP. Sites of distant recurrence and clinical outcomes in patients with metastatic triple-negative breast cancer: high incidence of central nervous system metastases. Cancer. 2008;113(10):2638–45.
30. Niwińska A, Murawska M, Pogoda K. Breast cancer subtypes and response to systemic treatment after whole-brain radiotherapy in patients with brain metastases. Cancer. 2010;116(18):4238–47.
31. Debien V, De Caluwé A, Wang X, et al. Immunotherapy in breast cancer: an overview of current strategies and perspectives. npj Breast Cancer. 2023;9(1):7.
32. Bardia A, Hurvitz SA, Tolaney SM, et al. Sacituzumab Govitecan in Metastatic Triple-Negative Breast Cancer. N Engl J Med. 2021;384:1529–41.
33. Copson ER, Maishman TC, Tapper WJ, et al. Germline BRCA mutation and outcome in young-onset breast cancer (POSH): a prospective cohort study. Lancet Oncol. 2018;19(2):169–80.
34. Robson M, Im S-A, Senkus E, et al. Olaparib for metastatic breast Cancer in patients with a germline *BRCA* mutation. N Engl J Med. 2017;377(6):523–33.
35. Tutt A, Tovey H, Cheang MCU, et al. Carboplatin in BRCA1/2-mutated and triple-negative breast cancer BRCAness subgroups: the TNT Trial. Nat Med. 2018;24(5):628–37
36. Tutt ANJ, Garber JE, Kaufman B, et al. Adjuvant Olaparib for Patients with BRCA1 - or BRCA2 -Mutated Breast Cancer. N Engl J Med. 2021;384:2394−2405.
37. Eisenhauer EA, Therasse P, Bogaerts J, et al. New response evaluation criteria in solid tumours: revised RECIST guideline (version 1.1). Eur J Cancer. 2009;45(2):228–47.

Radiological Imaging of Breast Cancer

4

Parveen Gulati and Narainder K. Gupta

Contents

4.1 Introduction

The decreasing morbidity and mortality due to breast cancer are in no small part due to early detection, staging, and post-treatment follow-up with imaging. This chapter discuss the role of various imaging modalities in breast cancer screening, diagnosis, staging, response assessment, and their various advantages and disadvantages. Essential to know normal variants, artifacts, and some clinical pearls are also emphasized.

P. Gulati
Gulati Imaging Institute, Delhi, India

N. K. Gupta (✉)
Department of Radiology, Hospital of the University of Pennsylvania, Philadelphia, PA, USA
e-mail: Narainder.Gupta@pennmedicine.upenn.edu

4.2   Screening and Diagnosis

A combination of clinical and radiological evaluation of the breast is essential. Screening guidelines for breast cancer differ from organization to organization. The Society Of Breast Imaging (SBI) and American College of Radiology (ACR) recommend annual mammography for women of average risk after the age of 40 years until life expectancy is <5–7 years on the basis of age or comorbid conditions or when abnormal results would not be acted upon due to age or comorbid factors. Women at high-risk start screening sooner, but at no less than 25 years [1].

4.2.1   Mammography

Mammography is the only known modality to decrease mortality from breast cancer via timely detection thus allowing treatment at an early stage. While it may lead to over diagnosis and over treatment, the benefits are found to be higher.

Standard craniocaudal and mediolateral oblique views are obtained with the breasts pulled away and compressed between two sheets of glass via exposure to low-dose X-rays. Hyperdense, spiculated, irregular masses, microcalcifications, architectural distortion, duct dilation, focal asymmetry, and small densities include some findings suspicious for malignancy (Fig. 4.1). Strict quality control and standardized reporting, usually following the BIRADS classification system, are essential. Core needle biopsy and needle localization of abnormalities can also be done under mammography guidance wherever required.

However, mammography does suffer from its own set of limitations. The compression is not only a source of great discomfort but also causes tissue overlap and may lead to a missed malignancy. This is an even bigger hazard in dense breast tissue in young females [2].

The advent of digital tomosynthesis mammography solves many of these problems—it allows a 3D reconstruction of breast tissue—increasing sensitivity and improving lesion characterization, especially in dense breasts. It is also more comfortable for the patients and has been shown to decrease the number of callbacks. The radiation exposure may, however, be slightly higher. While promising, this is currently not used as a screening tool on its own, but in combination with conventional mammography.

Computer-Aided Diagnosis has gained a stronghold in mammography by virtue of its ability to bring the most inconspicuous of findings of potential concern into focus thus acting as an extra layer of scrutiny before a final diagnosis, thus aiding in diagnosis at an earlier stage. It has also been suggested that it may be potentially advantageous, compared to conventional digital mammography, in women with denser breasts [3]. Owing to its success as a screening tool, this has been a constantly evolving field. Further advances like Contrast-Enhanced Digital Mammography and attempts to lower radiation exposure add further potential to this modality [4].

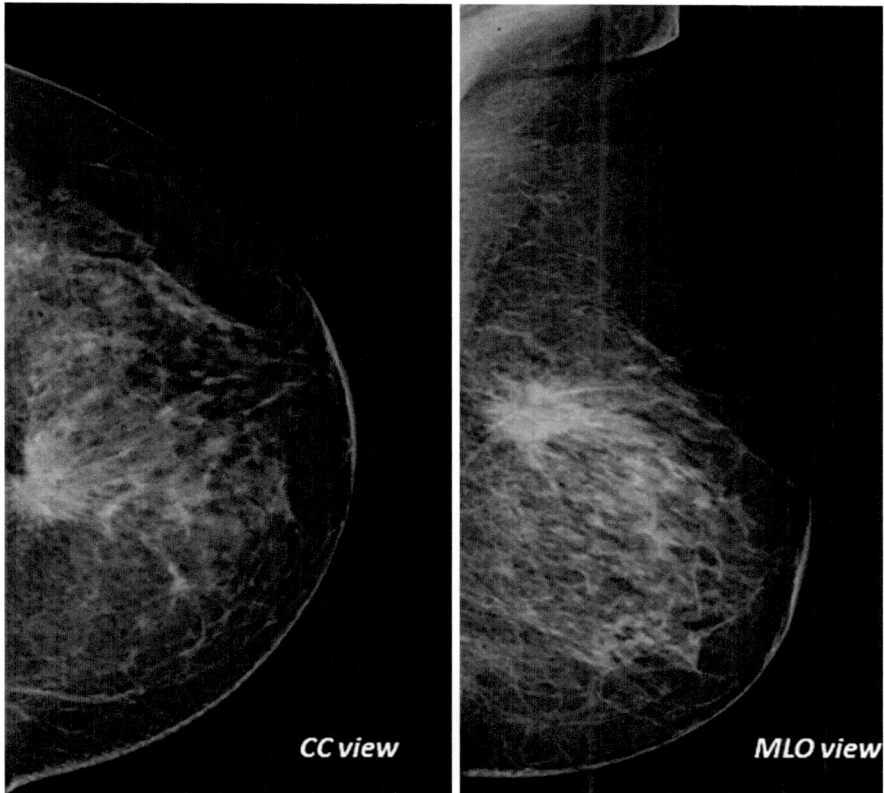

Fig. 4.1   X-RAY mammogram of breast showing an irregular, spiculated, high density mass lesion in the right breast. BIRADS 5. *CC* cranio-caudal, *MLO* mediolateral oblique

4.2.2   USG

With significant changes in technology including the development of high frequency probes, enhanced contrast resolution, harmonic imaging and panoramic views among others, ultrasonography has become indispensable in the evaluation of a breast lump. A high-resolution, real-time, linear-array, broad-bandwidth transducer operating at the highest frequency possible for optimum penetration, but at least 12 MHz, should be used for optimum contrast and spatial resolution [5, 6]. Reporting is usually done as per BIRADS-US. The recommended indications for Breast USG are mentioned in Table 4.1. The characteristic features of breast malignancy are mentioned in Table 4.2.

Colour Doppler sonography can be a good predictor of malignancy if used as an adjunct to other features, but does not have high predictive values when used on its own. However, blood flow in a known tumor corresponds well with tumor aggressiveness and grade and may be used to monitor treatment response. Doppler

Table 4.1 Indications of breast USG

Further evaluation of suspected abnormalities detected on other modalities
Axillary lymph node assessment
Follow up of lesions
Supplement to mammography screening in certain high risk populations with contraindications to, or no access to, MRI
Guidance for interventional procedures
Evaluation of implants and their complications
Planning of radiation therapy

Table 4.2 Characteristics of benign vs. malignant lesions on USG [7]

Benign	Malignant (Fig. 4.2)
Smooth, well circumscribed	Spiculation
Hyperechoic, isoechoic, or mildly hypoechoic	Taller than wider
Thin echogenic capsule	Angular margins
Ellipsoid shape, wider than taller	Shadowing
Three or fewer gentle lobulations	Branching pattern
No malignant findings	Hypoechogenicity
	Calcifications
	Duct extension
	Microlobulations

Fig. 4.2 Sono-mammogram of the right breast showing an irregular, heterogenous hypoechoic mass measuring about 13 × 16 × 19 mm, highly suspicious of a mitotic lesion – BIRADS 5. Core biopsy confirmed an adenocarcinoma

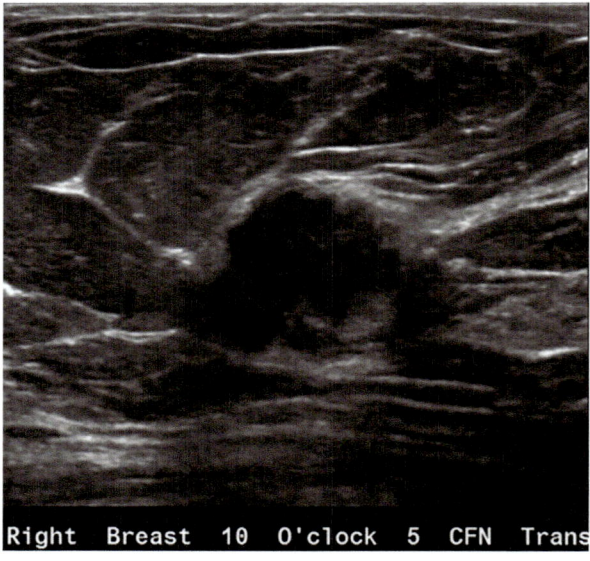

Right Breast 10 O'clock 5 CFN Trans

sonography is particularly useful for the characterization of solid or cystic lesions and for the detection of inflammation [8].

Quantitative measurement of tissue elasticity with sono-elastography adds another level of detail to breast ultrasound and increases the specificity. It has been shown to provide additional clarification especially for BIRADS-US 3 and 4 lesions.

With wider availability, lack of radiation exposure, and multiple technological advances, USG is fast gaining merit in breast evaluation. However, it does have a higher false-positive rate than mammography, is unable to detect microcalcifications and remains heavily operator dependent. Automated Breast USG has been shown to be potentially advantageous in preoperative assessment of breast cancer, especially pure DCIS and eliminated inter-observer variability [9, 10]. However, it can potentially miss smaller benign lesions [11].

4.2.3 MRI

Breast MRI is a widely used ancillary tool for the early detection and preoperative surgical planning of cancer (Table 4.3). It is usually performed on a 1.5 or preferably 3.0 Tesla magnet with a dedicated breast coil. Proper positioning is essential. Scanning slice thickness should be a maximum of 3 mm and resolution should be 1 mm or less. Imaging protocol should include pre- and dynamic post-contrast sequence and preferably Diffusion Weighted imaging and spectroscopy. Fat suppression is essential in contrast-enhanced breast imaging. The evaluation includes lesion characterization (Table 4.4), enhancement pattern with special emphasis on wash-in washout pattern, diffusion restriction, if any, and choline peak on spectroscopy.

Table 4.3 Common indications of breast MRI

- High-risk patients, e.g., BRCA1/2 personal history or family history, history of radiation, history of cancer syndromes, prior diagnosis of atypia/lobular carcinoma in situ/breast cancer.
- Preoperative evaluation of tumor for size, extent, multifocality, and multicentricity.
- Post-surgery to differentiate between recurrence or scar tissue.
- Post-chemotherapy to check for a response.
- Breast implants, evaluation of rupture.

Table 4.4 Findings suspicious of malignancy on MRI (Fig. 4.3)

Irregular or spiculated margins
Rim-like enhancement
Heterogenous internal enhancement and enhancing internal septa
Type III curve on dynamic contrast
Nipple changes such as retraction, inversion
Skin changes such as invasion, retraction, thickening, and edema
Lymphadenopathy
Pre-contrast high ductal signal
Obliteration of the fat plane and muscle enhancement

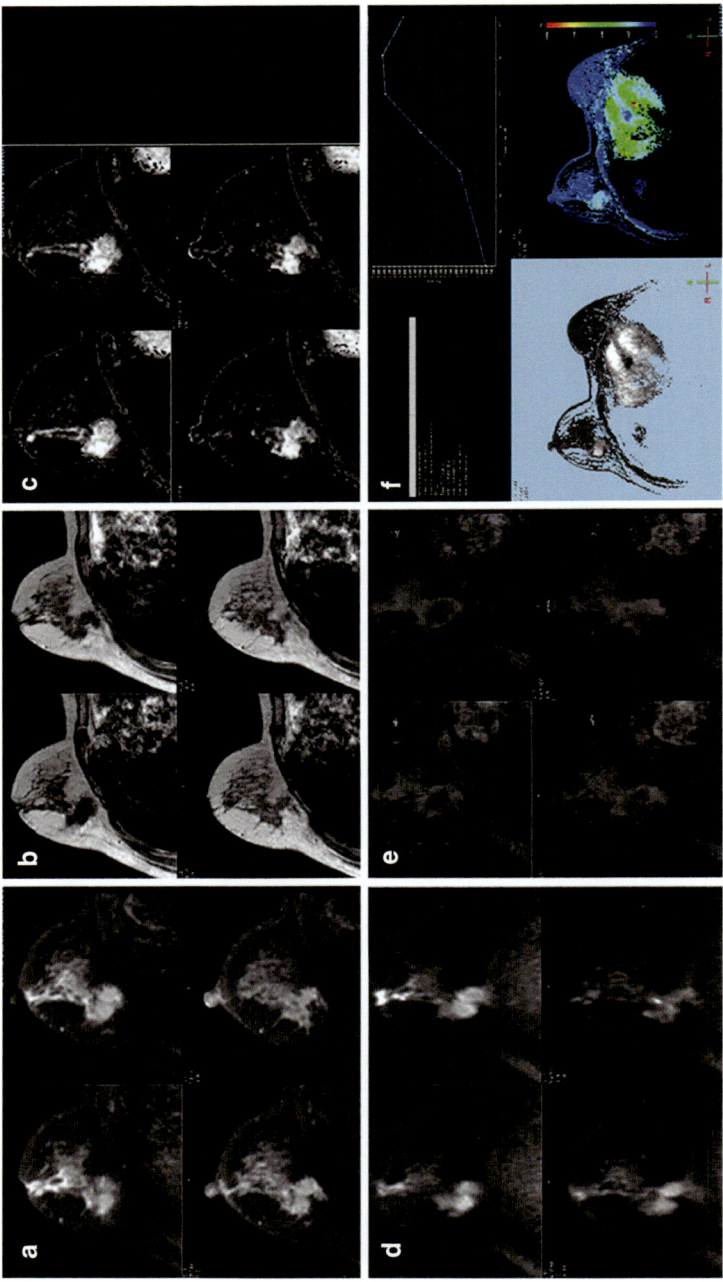

Fig. 4.3 FATSAT T2 (**a**) & T1 (**b**) weighted images showing an irregular lobulated mass with spiculated margins in the right breast, showing hyperintense signal on T2 FATSAT and low intense signal on T1 images. The mass shows extension upto the nipple anteriorly and to chest wall posteriorly. The mass shows restricted diffusion evidenced by bright signal on DWI (**c**) and low-intense signal on ADC images. (**d**). Post contrast scans (**e**) reveal dense enhancement of the mass with dynamic perfusion scan (**f**) showing type III enhancment pattern --- all features are suggestive of a mitotic lesion (MR BIRAD 5)

It offers many advantages, e.g., the use of non-ionizing radiation, better 3D spatial resolution, detection of multicentricity and multifocality, better delineation of the extent of the tumor, and imaging of the breasts and chest wall together. In the event of a discrepancy in tumor measurements using different imaging modalities, MR imaging has been shown to be the most accurate [12]. It does, however, have a higher false-positive rate as benign lesions are also picked up well. Its cost, being resource and time intensive and being less tolerable to patients as compared to mammography or USG and difficulty in use with obese patients, or patients with metallic implants or other devices also make it prohibitive.

CAD for breast MRI is an area of rapid development and has been shown to have utility in the detection of tumor multifocality and extent. However, it is limited in its ability to detect LN status [13].

4.2.4   Thermography

Angiogenesis in a cancerous or precancerous lesion along with the increased metabolic rate can lead to elevated temperatures in the breast compared to the normal breast tissue. These changes in temperature can detect cancers and monitor early signs in a non-invasive, non-compressive manner that does not use radiation and is time efficient. The thermo biological grading system is used, but interpretation still depends, to a large extent, on the analyst. Moreover, it is not very effective at diagnosing malignancies at a depth. It shows great promise but is not used as an independent screening tool but in combination with mammography.

4.3   Staging of Breast Cancer

Diagnostic mammography with the routine craniocaudal and mediolateral oblique views is done with the addition of supplementary views as determined by the screening mammogram. MRI and US improve upon the staging. CT, PET/CT, and Bone Scan are used to detect metastasis (Figs. 4.4 and 4.5).

T1, T2, T3: AJCC's TNM Staging System defines stages T1, T2, and T3 as follows: T1-invasive tumors </= 20 mm, subdivided into T1mi (≤1 mm), T1a (>1 mm but ≤5 mm), T1b (>5 mm but ≤10 mm), and T1c (>10 mm but ≤20 mm), T2: 20–50 mm, and T3: >50 mm.

T4: T4 includes a tumor of any size with direct extension to the chest wall and/or to the skin (ulceration or skin nodules), including IBC. Contrast-enhanced breast MRI is the optimal modality for determining chest wall invasion the signs of which include obliteration of the fat plane and muscle enhancement.

Nodal Staging: Surgical evaluation with SLNB remains the definitive diagnosis for nodal metastasis, imaging serves to aid in planning ALND. Micro-metastases identification remains a limitation in imaging. US is the primary imaging modality for node status assessment. A suspicious USG finding with a high risk of axillary

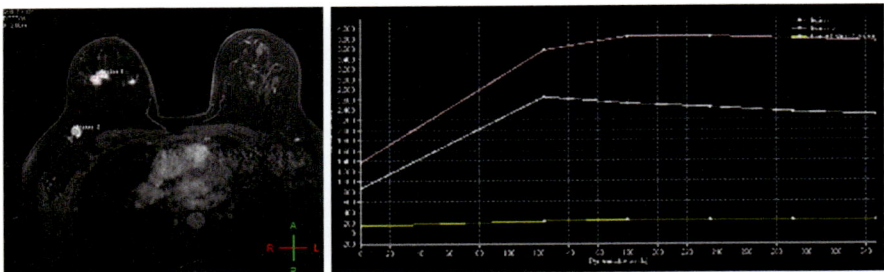

Fig. 4.4 45 year old lady showed a solitary spiculated lesion on X RAY mammogram, PLAN: Breast conservative surgery MR mammography reveals multiple enhancing lesions on contrast FAT SAT scans with dynamic scans showing type II/type III curve - multicentric mitotic lesion - MR findings changed the management

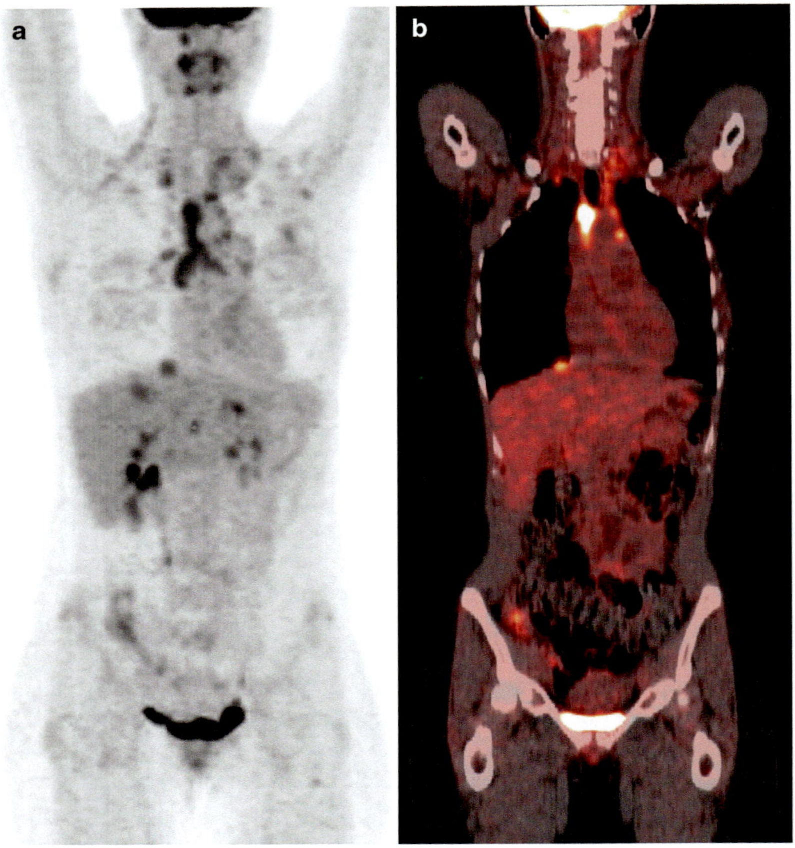

Fig. 4.5 PET-CT IMAGES (**a**, **b**) in a 32 years old follow up case of carcinoma breast showing metastatic adenopathy involving the mediastinum, chest wall and supra-clavicular regions, as well as likely metastatic involvement in a retroperitoneal lymph node. There are associated hypermetabolic hepatic lesions in segment 4, suggestive of metastatic disease

metastases warrants percutaneous procedures like US-FNA or US-CNB before a full ALND [14].

Metastasis: Distant metastases are most commonly seen in the bones, lungs, liver, and brain. High-risk asymptomatic patients—stage IIIA or higher and all symptomatic patients must undergo a complete workup for detecting metastasis. Chest radiography, abdominal US, CT, MRI, and PET/CT are usually used as per the treating physician's discretion as there is a lack of consensus regarding for whom and how screening for metastasis should ideally be done in spite of multiple guidelines. FDG-PET is usually recommended for recurrent or stage IV disease for the detection of metastases and occult disease. It has been shown to improve the staging and alter the therapeutic plan by detecting widespread disease with a high sensitivity and specificity. However, it often fails to detect osteoblastic lesions, which may be more easily picked up by bone scintigraphy.

4.4 Response Assessment and Surveillance

There is currently no single ideal imaging modality for surveillance and monitoring.

Mammography remains the mainstay of surveillance with the ASCO recommending that the first after-treatment mammogram be done 1 year after the initial mammogram that leads to diagnosis but not earlier than 6 months after definitive radiotherapy [15]. However, the intervals at which to repeat it are still debated. The sensitivity and specificity of mammography are greatly decreased due to postoperative scars and post-radiation changes.

US has a high sensitivity for detecting ipsilateral or contralateral recurrences and is vital in the assessment of axial lymph nodes and the chest wall, which is a common site of recurrence. However, its role in post-treatment surveillance is not yet established.

Breast MRI is found to be superior to other imaging modalities in its ability to pick up abnormalities in post-treatment sites and differentiate new tumors from scar tissue. It also has been shown to have the maximum correlation with pathological disease extent and in prediction of residual disease after neoadjuvant chemotherapy [16].

FDG-PET has a high sensitivity but low specificity in the case of neoadjuvant therapy. However, it does hold merit for the detection of recurrence—whether isolated or widespread.

There remains a lack of clear guidelines for the use of different modalities, but they have all been shown to be powerful tools in their own right.

4.5 Radiotherapy Planning

An optimal target volume definition (TVD) is essential in radiotherapy so as to ensure that the prescribed dose is delivered to tumor cells while minimizing radiation to the healthy tissue.

CT is currently the modality of choice for obtaining the planning scan owing to its excellent geometrical accuracy, the provision of electron density information that is necessary for planning tissue dose calculations and its ability to acquire information in a very short span of time (of the order of seconds). It is also easier to position patients in the required RT position. However, it does suffer from the inability to discriminate well between adjacent tissue of similar attenuation unless separated by fat, bone, or air.

Although the role of MRI in radiotherapy planning is rapidly expanding, its position is dubious in RTP for breast cancer. MRI planning scans need to be performed in the suboptimal supine position, a disadvantage further compounded by the deformable nature of breasts. The target volume obtained is found to be inaccurate, irregular, and speckled. The use of MR-CT co-registration also has not been found to be significantly beneficial [17].

4.6   Artifacts on Imaging

Recognition of important common artifacts, their minimization and correction are essential for obtaining optimal image quality.

On digital mammography, artifacts may be due to patient, hardware, or software factors. Artifacts rooted in patient factors include motion artifacts, antiperspirant artifacts which may mimic calcifications and artifacts due to breasts that compress to less than 2 cm thickness that may cause inclusion of the paddle edges. In order to minimize these, patients must always be advised to be absolutely still, exposure time should be minimal, compression may be increased and the breast-axilla region must be clean. Hardware-related artifacts include collimator misalignment, detector-associated artifacts like ghosting and gouging, field inhomogeneity at quality control imaging, underexposure, grid lines or grid misplacement, and vibration effects. High-density artifact, breast-within-a-breast, loss of edge or the appearance of vertical processing bars all occur due to software defects [18].

On MRI, motion artifacts, wraparound artifacts, inhomogeneous fat saturation, susceptibility artifacts, or inadequate exposure may deteriorate image quality. Misregistration artifacts are peculiar to subtraction imaging and occur when there is relative motion between two images to be subtracted [19].

4.7   Essential to Remember

1. During screening, always compare with previous mammograms.
2. Always look for internal mammary node metastasis as it affects the staging, prognosis as well as radiation therapy planning.
3. Pectoralis muscle involvement does not alter staging, but impacts surgical planning and is thus important to note.

4. Always look for multifocal and multicentric diseases as they affect the surgical plan.
5. MRI protocol should always include pre and dynamic contrast sequences and preferably diffusion and spectroscopy.
6. Whenever in doubt with one modality do not hesitate to confirm the findings on another modality before deciding on the management.

References

1. Lee CH, Dershaw DD, Kopans D, Evans P, Monsees B, Monticciolo D, et al. Breast cancer screening with imaging: recommendations from the Society of Breast Imaging and the ACR on the use of mammography, breast MRI, breast ultrasound, and other technologies for the detection of clinically occult breast cancer. J Am Coll Radiol. 2010;7(1):18–27.
2. Shetty MK. Screening for breast cancer with mammography: current status and an overview. Indian J Surg Oncol. 2010;1(3):218–23.
3. Hadjiiski L, Sahiner B, Chan HP. Advances in computer-aided diagnosis for breast cancer. Curr Opin Obstet Gynecol. 2006;18(1):64–70.
4. Helvie MA. Digital mammography imaging: breast tomosynthesis and advanced applications. Radiol Clin N Am. 2010;48(5):917–29.
5. ACR Practice Parameter for the Performance of a Breast Ultrasound Examination. 2016.
6. Gokhale S. Ultrasound characterization of breast masses. Indian J Radiol Imaging. 2009;19(3):242–7.
7. Stavros AT, Thickman D, Rapp CL, Dennis MA, Parker SH, Sisney GA. Solid breast nodules: use of sonography to distinguish between benign and malignant lesions. Radiology. 1995;196(1):123–34.
8. Busilacchi P, Draghi F, Preda L, Ferranti C. Has color Doppler a role in the evaluation of mammary lesions? J Ultrasound. 2012;15(2):93–8.
9. Berg WA, Bandos AI, Mendelson EB, Lehrer D, Jong RA, Pisano ED. Ultrasound as the primary screening test for breast cancer: analysis from ACRIN 6666. J Natl Cancer Inst. 2016;108(4):djv367.
10. Shin HJ, Kim HH, Cha JH. Current status of automated breast ultrasonography. Ultrasonography. 2015;34(3):165–72.
11. Jeh SK, Kim SH, Choi JJ, Jung SS, Choe BJ, Park S, et al. Comparison of automated breast ultrasonography to handheld ultrasonography in detecting and diagnosing breast lesions. Acta Radiol. 2016;57(2):162–9.
12. Boetes C, Mus RD, Holland R, Barentsz JO, Strijk SP, Wobbes T, et al. Breast tumors: comparative accuracy of MR imaging relative to mammography and US for demonstrating extent. Radiology. 1995;197(3):743–7.
13. Song SE, Seo BK, Cho KR, Woo OH, Son GS, Kim C, et al. Computer-aided detection (CAD) system for breast MRI in assessment of local tumor extent, nodal status, and multifocality of invasive breast cancers: preliminary study. Cancer Imaging. 2015;15:1.
14. Ecanow JS, Abe H, Newstead GM, Ecanow DB, Jeske JM. Axillary staging of breast cancer: what the radiologist should know. Radiographics. 2013;33(6):1589–612.
15. Khatcheressian JL, Hurley P, Bantug E, Esserman LJ, Grunfeld E, Halberg F, et al. Breast cancer follow-up and management after primary treatment: American Society of Clinical Oncology clinical practice guideline update. J Clin Oncol. 2013;31(7):961–5.
16. Manal Hamisa ND, Yosef R, Zakeria F, Hammed Q. Role of breast ultrasound, mammography, magnetic resonance imaging and diffusion weighted imaging in predicting

pathologic response of breast cancer after neoadjuvant chemotherapy. Egypt J Radiol Nucl Med. 2015;46(1):245–57.

17. Schmidt MA, Payne GS. Radiotherapy planning using MRI. Phys Med Biol. 2015;60(22):R323–61.

18. Ayyala RS, Chorlton M, Behrman RH, Kornguth PJ, Slanetz PJ. Digital mammographic artifacts on full-field systems: what are they and how do I fix them? Radiographics. 2008;28(7):1999–2008.

19. Ojeda-Fournier H, Choe KA, Mahoney MC. Recognizing and interpreting artifacts and pitfalls in MR imaging of the breast. Radiographics. 2007;27(Suppl 1):S147–64.

FDG PET/CT in Breast Cancer

5

Rakesh Kumar, Ravi Kant Gupta, Krishan Kant Agarwal, and Siraj Yusuf

Contents

5.1 Introduction

Positron emission tomography (PET) allows the assessment of biomarkers characteristic of a neoplastic cell or related to its environment. The cellular biomarkers of breast cancer reveal changes in glucose metabolism, amino acid transport and protein synthesis, DNA synthesis and cell proliferation, receptor expression (epidermal

R. Kumar (✉) · R. K. Gupta · K. K. Agarwal
Diagnostic Nuclear Medicine Division, Department of Nuclear Medicine, All India Institute of Medical Sciences, New Delhi, India

S. Yusuf
Department of Diagnostic Radiology, The Royal Marsden NHS Foundation Trust, London, UK

© The Author(s), under exclusive license to Springer Nature Switzerland AG 2023
R. Kumar et al. (eds.), *PET/CT in Breast Cancer*, Clinicians' Guides to Radionuclide Hybrid Imaging, https://doi.org/10.1007/978-3-031-29590-4_5

growth factor receptor, estrogen, and progesterone receptors), and induction of apoptosis. Variations in tumor blood flow, vascular permeability, and neoangiogenesis, along with hypoxia are biological processes that take place in the tissues surrounding cancer [1]. The main advantage of combined PET/CT (Positron Emission Tomography fused with Computed Tomography) imaging is its ability to accurately correlate abnormal metabolic changes detected on PET imaging to anatomic structures defined at CT imaging. The most commonly assessed oncological biomarker with PET is [18F] 2-deoxy-2-fluoro-d-glucose (18F-FDG) uptake. It is showing increasing usefulness in the distinction between malignant and benign lesions, in disease staging, re-staging, therapy planning, and monitoring [2].

5.2   Primary Diagnosis and Staging

PET/CT has revealed a good diagnostic accuracy in visualizing both primary cancer and metastatic lesions. PET as a diagnostic approach at the first presentation of a breast mass did not show a higher sensitivity than mammography and ultrasonography except in some particular situations. PET/CT has a role in initial staging of patients with locally advanced (LABC) invasive or inflammatory breast cancer when conventional staging studies (e.g., CT or bone scan) are equivocal or suspicious, especially in the setting of locally advanced or metastatic disease. ^{18}F-FDG PET/CT is a sensitive and specific imaging modality for identifying distant metastases in patients with LABC missed by conventional imaging. The usefulness of PET/CT for lymph node staging in breast cancer patients is limited because of the lack of sensitivity of PET/CT in depicting the small metastases spread to axillary lymph nodes. Sonographically guided FNA was found to be an excellent diagnostic tool for preoperative evaluation of the axillary lymph node (ALN) status [3]. Combined evaluation of ALNs by 18F-FDG PET/CT with that of sonography and sonographically guided fine-needle aspiration (FNA) modalities may be more complementary than the use of a single modality. Therefore, breast cancer patients with FDG-positive uptake should directly undergo ALN dissection. On the contrary, those cases without FDG uptake in the axilla should be examined with sonographically guided fine-needle aspiration (FNA) in order to select candidates for ALND (Figs. 5.1, 5.2, and 5.3).

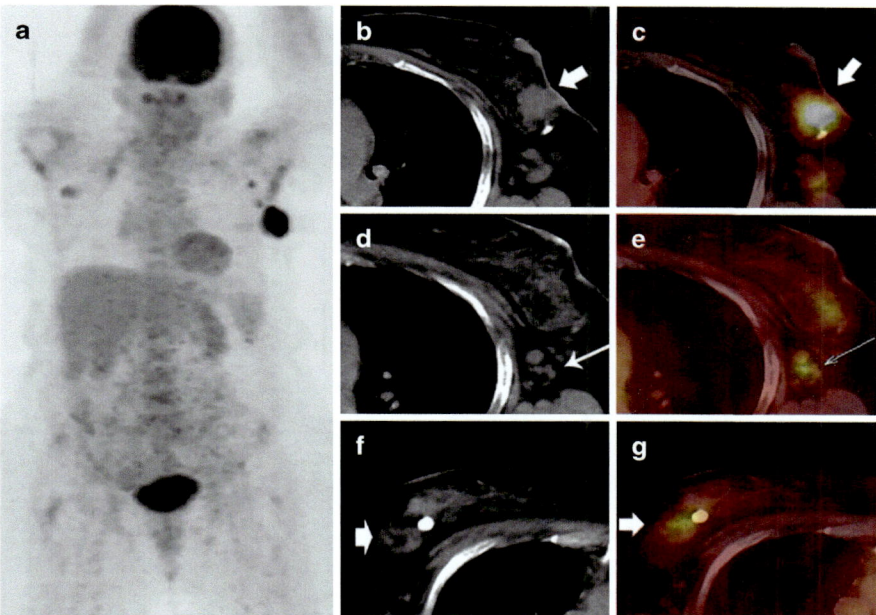

Fig. 5.1 A 77-year-old female with left breast carcinoma was referred for FDG PET/CT scan for staging. MIP image (**a**) shows primary pathology in left breast with left axillary lymph nodes metastases. (**b, c**) In axial CT (**b**) and PET/CT (**c**) images, FDG avid soft tissue density mass is seen with macro calcification in the lower outer quadrant of left breast involving overlying skin suggestive of primary site (arrows). Multiple left axillary lymph nodes with tracer uptake were noted in transaxial CT (**d**) and PET/CT (**e**) images (arrows). Also noted macro calcification with nodularity in right breast parenchyma with tracer uptake in axial CT (**f**) and PET/CT (**g**) images. The patient was advised for further evaluation to rule out second primary in the right breast

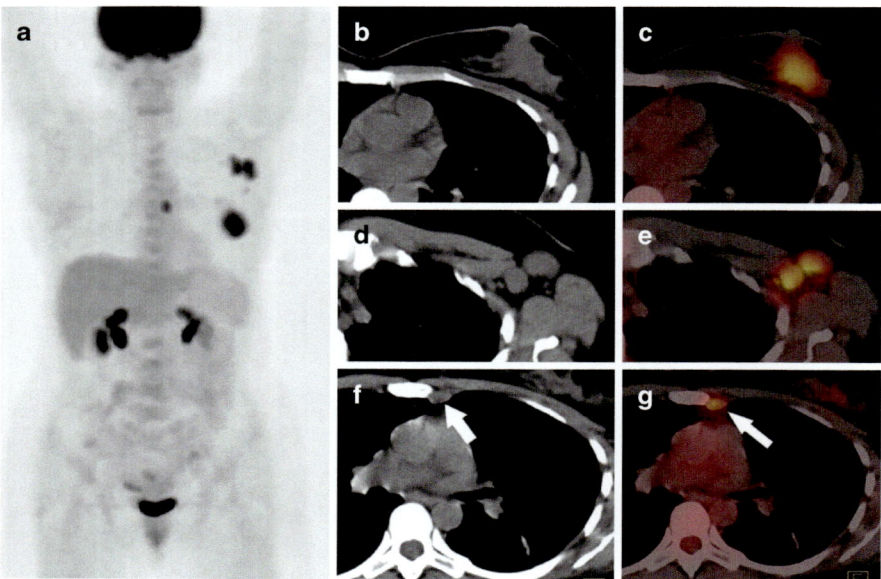

Fig. 5.2 A 38-year-old female presented with left breast carcinoma. MIP image (**a**) shows primary pathology in left breast with left axillary and left internal mammary lymph nodes metastases. Transaxial CT (**b**) and PET/CT (**c**) show FDG avid soft tissue density mass in retroareolar region of left breast suggestive of the primary site. Transaxial CT (**d**) and PET/CT (**e**) images show FDG avid left axillary lymph nodes consistent with metastatic involvement. Also noted left internal mammary lymph nodes with increased tracer uptake in transaxial CT (**f**) and PET/CT (**g**) images

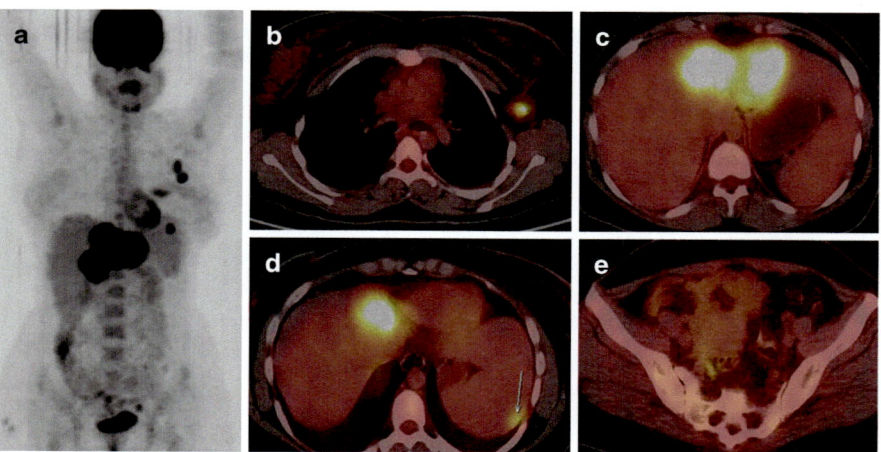

Fig. 5.3 A 26-year-old female with left breast carcinoma was referred for FDG PET/CT scan for restaging after lumpectomy. MIP (**a**) and axial PET/CT (**b–d**) images show metabolically active left axillary lymph nodes (**b**) and subcapsular liver and spleen lesions (**c, d**). In view of subcapsular liver and spleen lesions with a right adnexal cyst in transaxial PET/CT (**e**) image, patient was advised CA-125 correlation to rule out second primary in the adnexa

5.3   Response Assessment

In LABC, standard treatment consists of neo-adjuvant chemotherapy, usually anthracycline-based, or more recently with taxanes or endocrine therapy, followed by mastectomy with axillary lymphadenectomy and irradiation of the chest wall. The aim of such neo-adjuvant systemic therapy is to eliminate occult distant metastases and to downstage tumor load prior to surgery, rendering previously inoperable breast cancer resectable, and/or to enable breast-conserving surgery and sentinel node biopsy instead of axillary lymph node dissection [4]. 18F-FDG PET/CT has reasonable sensitivity in evaluating response to neoadjuvant chemotherapy in breast cancer; however, the specificity is relatively low. The combination of other imaging methods with 18F-FDG PET/CT is recommended. Early decrease in FDG uptake, e.g., after only one course of chemotherapy, can predict pathological response. Furthermore, persistent decline in FDG uptake, demonstrated by serial scans, may also predict (complete) clinical and pathological responses. In contrast, persisting focal 18F-FDG uptake is likely to be indicative of either only partial pathological response or poor clinical outcome [5–7].

In patients with metastatic breast cancer, the effectiveness of chemotherapy can be evaluated with 18F-FDG PET than with conventional imaging. Sequential 18F-FDG PET performed at baseline and after initiation of treatment allowed prediction of response as early as after the first cycle of chemotherapy [8]. The use of 18F-FDG PET findings as a surrogate endpoint for predicting therapy response offers improved patient care by individualizing treatment and avoiding ineffective chemotherapy (Figs. 5.4, 5.5, 5.6, 5.7, and 5.8).

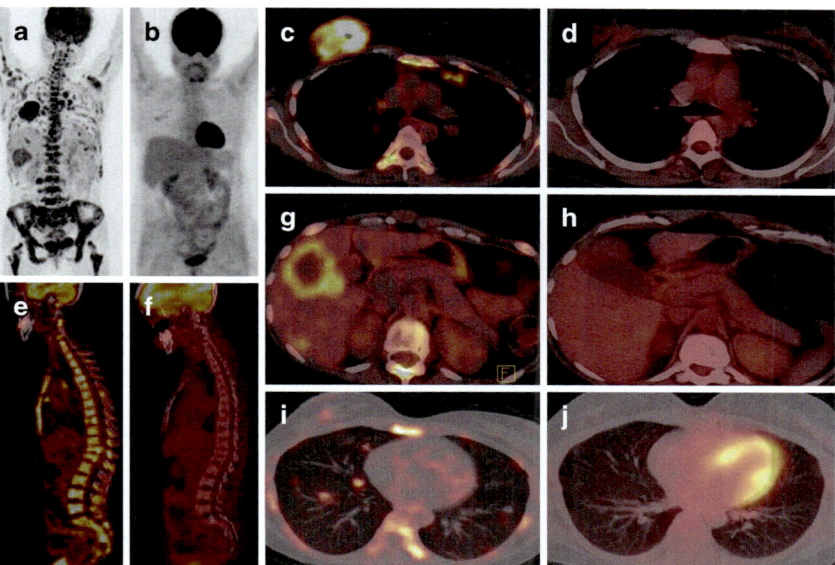

Fig. 5.4   A 33-year-old female with right breast carcinoma underwent FDG PET/CT scan for response evaluation after neoadjuvant chemotherapy. In pretreatment FDG PET MIP (**a**), transaxial PET/CT (**c**, **g**, **i**) and sagittal (**e**) images showed primary malignant pathology in right breast with right axillary lymph nodes, liver (**g**), bilateral lungs (**i**), and skeletal (**e**) metastases. After chemotherapy, there is a near complete metabolic response in MIP (**b**), transaxial PET/CT (**d**, **h**, **j**), and sagittal (**f**) images

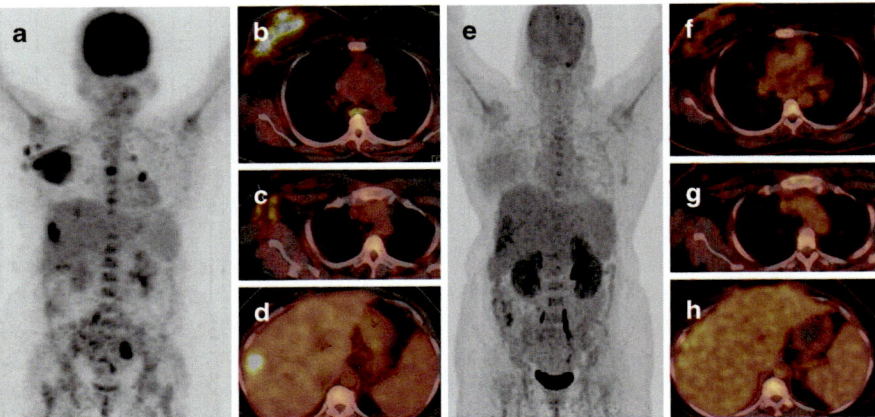

Fig. 5.5 A 42-year-old female with right breast carcinoma was referred for FDG PET/CT scan for response evaluation after neoadjuvant chemotherapy. Pretreatment MIP (**a**) and transaxial PET/CT (**b–d**) images show metabolically active primary pathology in right breast (**b**) with right axillary lymph nodes (**c**) and liver metastases (**d**). Post chemotherapy, there is decrease in size and tracer uptake of right breast lesion (**f**) and liver lesion (**h**) with decrease in number, size, and tracer uptake of right axillary lymph nodes (**g**) can be well appreciated on post-treatment MIP images (**e**) suggestive of partial response

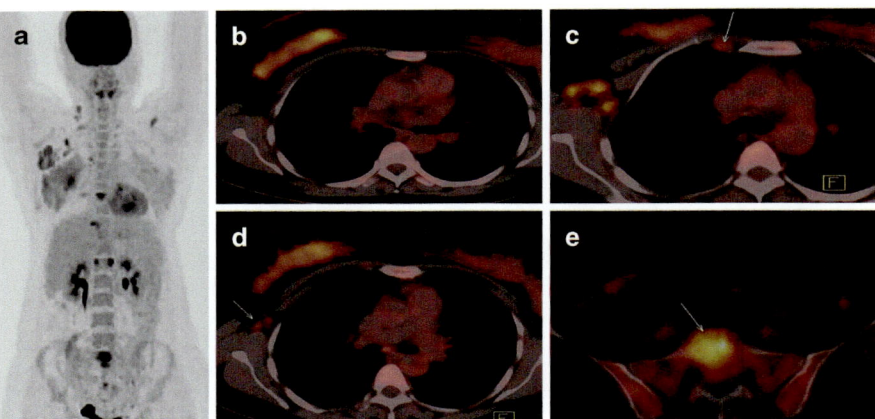

Fig. 5.6 A 30-year-old female with invasive ductal carcinoma of right breast was referred for FDG PET/CT scan for response evaluation after chemoradiotherapy. Pretreatment FDG PET/CT (**a**) shows metabolically active primary pathology in right breast (**b**) with right axillary (**c, d**), and right internal mammary (**c**) lymph nodes and multiple skeletal metastases (**e**). Post-treatment study (**f**) shows resolution of primary right breast lesion (**g**) and right axillary (**h, i**) and right internal mammary (**h**) lymph nodes and skeletal lesions (**j**) suggestive of complete metabolic response

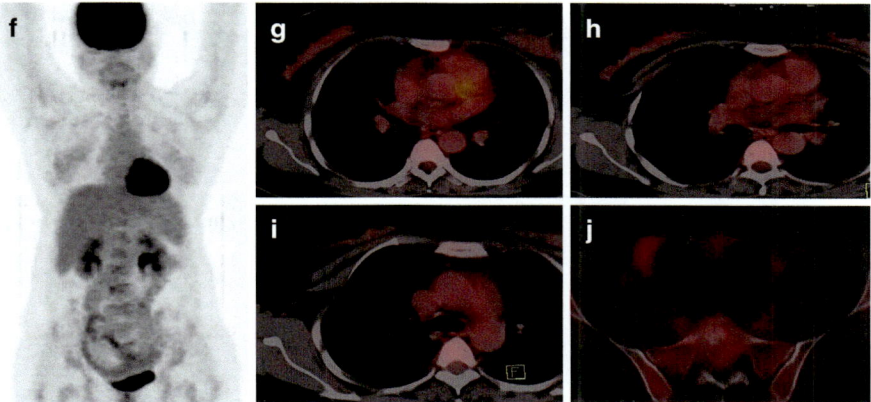

Fig. 5.6 (Continued)

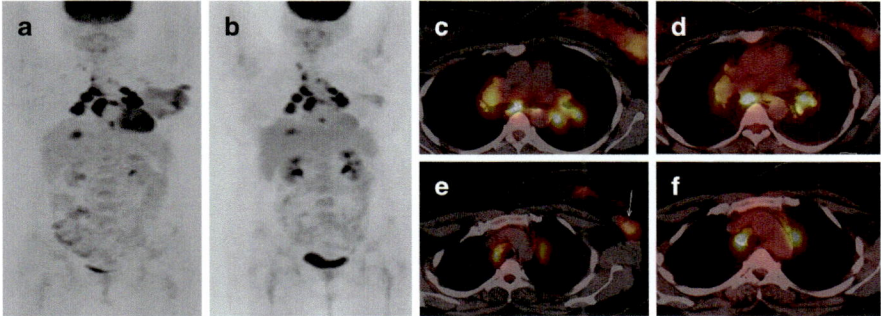

Fig. 5.7 A 35-year-old female with left breast carcinoma was referred for FDG PET/CT scan for response evaluation after neoadjuvant chemotherapy. Pretreatment FDG PET/CT shows (MIP-**a**, axial **c**, **e**) metabolically active primary pathology in left breast (**c**) with left axillary lymph nodes metastases (**e**). Also noted FDG avid bilateral hilar and mediastinal lymphadenopathy in transaxial PET/CT images (**c**, **e**). Post-chemotherapy PET/CT shows regression in size and tracer uptake of left breast lesion and left axillary lymph nodes in MIP (**b**) and transaxial PET/CT (**d**, **f**) images suggestive of partial response. However, bilateral hilar and mediastinal lymphadenopathy shows no interval regression in metabolic activity (**c–f**) suggestive of benign pathology

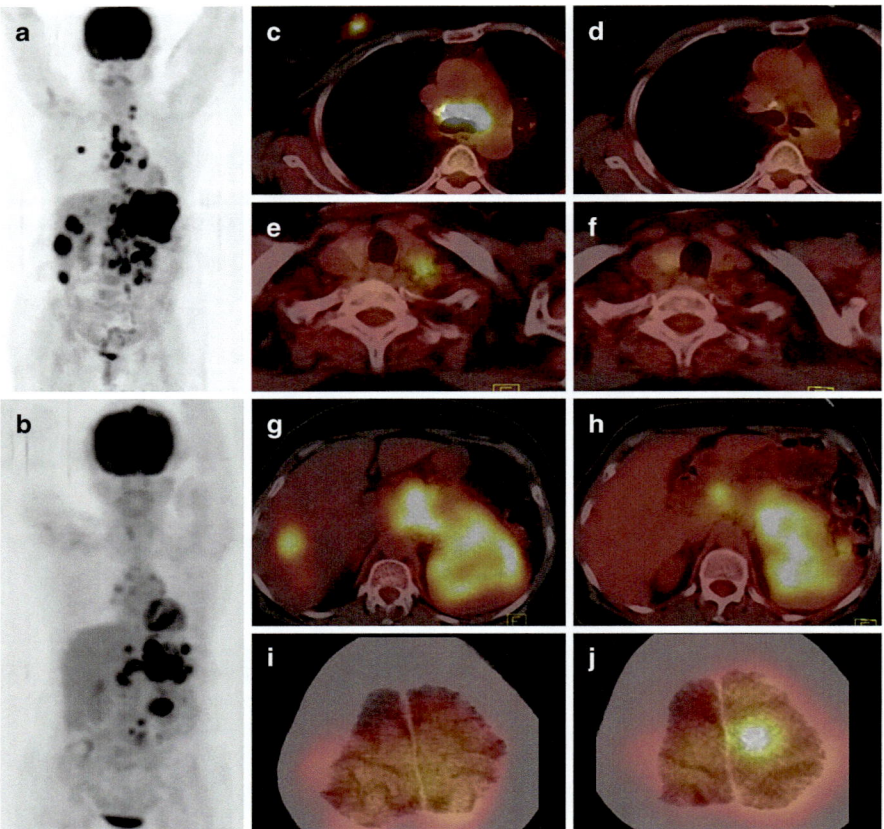

Fig. 5.8 A 63-year-old female with invasive ductal carcinoma in right breast was referred for FDG PET/CT scan for response evaluation after chemotherapy. Baseline MIP (**a**) and transaxial PET/CT (**c, e, g, i**) images show metabolically active primary pathology in right breast (**c**) with left supraclavicular (**e**), mediastinal and retroperitoneal lymph nodes, and liver metastases (**g**). Post-chemotherapy, there is resolution of right breast lesion (**b, d**), left supraclavicular (**f**) and mediastinal lymph nodes and liver lesion (**h**), however, there is the appearance of new brain metastases suggestive of disease progression (**i, j**)

5.4   Radiotherapy Planning

PET scans before, during, and after treatment may provide information that is useful for managing patients undergoing radiation therapy. A pre-treatment PET/CT study allows not only to evaluate metabolic tumor activity but also treatment planning. PET/CT has been used to assess the therapeutic response to radiation therapy. ^{18}F-FDG PET/CT can identify changes in glucose uptake after treatment and may prove to be a better indicator of a favorable response to therapy. However, it may be important to differentiate between a decrease in FDG uptake and the complete absence of FDG uptake. Post-treatment normalization of FDG uptake will probably be a good prognostic sign. Usually, a PET tumor complete response will be predictive of improved survival.

A major problem of post-radiation therapy PET/CT is that normal tissues can manifest radiotherapy toxicity to different degrees. Some tissues will demonstrate toxicity in a few days. These tissues are bone marrow, gonads, lymph nodes, salivary glands, gastrointestinal tract, larynx, and skin [9]. Other tissues demonstrate radiation damage in weeks to months, and some examples are lung, liver, kidney, spinal cord, and brain. Because of these effects, significantly increased FDG uptake can be seen in selected soft tissue regions that are irradiated. Radiotherapy may induce early acute inflammatory hypermetabolism on PET that is likely related to healing of tissues damaged by radiation. This effect will of course depend on the radiosensitivity of the normal tissue being irradiated. For example, increased FDG uptake may be found at 12–16 months after treatment. Normal tissue activity inflammatory responses are at maximum at about 6 months, but can be seen for at least 1 year [10, 11].

5.5 Normal Variants and Artifacts

The normal distribution of 18F-FDG reflects glucose metabolism. Physiological FDG uptake occurs in brain due to its obligate glucose dependence. The genitourinary tract also shows intense activity due to urinary clearance of 18F-FDG. Variable activity occurs in the heart, gastrointestinal tract, salivary glands, and testes. The uterus may show endometrial uptake depending on the menstrual cycle stage.

5.5.1 Benign Variants

The skeletal muscles may show prominent uptake due to recent exertion. Another common variant is 18F-FDG accumulation in supraclavicular region so-called "brown fat." This variant occurs more commonly in cold weather and cold patients. Brown fat contains adrenergic receptors that contribute to uptake in anxious patients.

5.5.2 Effects of Inflammation and Therapy

18F-FDG uptake is not specific for tumor. Increased activity can be seen in inflammation and infection, and the cause has been attributed to glycolytic activity in leukocytes. Infections such as pneumonia will have intense radiotracer accumulation. Inflammatory uptake in a lymph node or mass cannot be differentiated from malignancy. Therapy often results in an inflammatory response causing increased activity. Radiation therapy causes intense 18F-FDG uptake. PET/CT scan is delayed for 3 months radiotherapy-induced uptake may persist for many months. Chemotherapy may cause a lesion to show a transient apparent worsening. A delay in scanning of several weeks or until just before beginning the next chemotherapy cycle is currently recommended [12].

5.6   Artifacts

Attenuation-correction images may mistakenly show increased radiotracer activity when metal or dense-iodinated contrast is present. Areas of intense 18F-FDG activity, such as in the bladder and infiltration at the injection site, can cause a reconstruction artifact manifested by a band of artifactually decreased activity across the patient. Examining the nonattenuation-corrected images can lead to the correct interpretation.

A common artifact is caused by misregistration of PET and CT data due to respiration. Respiratory motion artifacts can also cause abnormal uptake from a lesion to appear in an incorrect location on the CT, particularly, for pathology near the diaphragm. Truncation artifact is thin linear bands of activity along the patient's axis on the maximum-intensity projection image and commonly occurs if the patient is large or imaged with arms at their sides. CT beam-hardening artifact is a common problem that affects the quality of the CT and fused PET/CT images. This can be minimized by moving the arms out of the field of view. Another common, subtle artifact is a thin horizontal band or seam perpendicular to the patient's axis from adjoining bed positions.

5.7   Advantages

PET/CT shows more accuracy than conventional imaging in the diagnosis of metastatic disease at cancer presentation (except for loco-regional lymph node invasion). In recurrent metastatic disease, PET/CT has high accuracy (around 90%) for the detection of metastatic disease and also shows good sensitivity in depiction of loco-regional recurrences [13]. During follow-up cases in asymptomatic patients with a progressive increase of tumor marker levels, PET/CT depicts high sensitivity (more than 90%) for the detection of occult recurrence [14–17].

5.8   Limitations/Pitfalls

PET/CT shows false-negative results in breast cancer with low metabolism (lobular carcinoma). PET/CT usefulness is related to the stage of disease. The use of PET/CT scanning is not indicated in the early stages of breast cancer. PET/CT has a high false-negative rate in detection of small (<1 cm) and/or low-grade lesions, the low sensitivity for detection of axillary nodal metastases [18]. Other limitations of 18F-FDG PET/CT in the follow-up of breast cancer patients include the relatively low detection rate of bone metastases, especially in case of sclerotic subtype. This limitation is overcome by radiopharmaceuticals like 18F-fluoride PET/CT which has both sensitive and specific for the detection of lytic and sclerotic bone metastases [19].

5.9   Sentinel Lymph Node

Axillary node status is a major prognostic factor in early-stage breast cancer. Sentinel lymph node dissection (SLND) is now standard axillary staging procedure for the determination of axillary lymph node status in breast cancer patients without clinically palpable axillary lymph nodes [20–23].

Sentinel lymph node (SLN) can be identified by blue dye or by radiotracer, or by both. When it is identified by radiotracer, the incision is made over the hottest spot visualized in the axilla. If blue dye is used, the incision is usually made about 1–2 cm below the hairline in the axilla [24, 25].

Badly chosen incision can cause difficulty in mapping intraoperative lymphatics, especially by use of blue dye method [24]. However, radioisotope-guided SLND can help in planning of incision for SLND guided by blue dye. Also, it can help to identify lymph node preoperatively by ultrasound.

Many radiopharmaceuticals have been used for the purpose of SLND. The commonly used agents are Tc-99 m sulfur colloid (SC), Tc-99 m nanocolloid, and Tc-99 m antimony trisulfide. As the particle sizes for sulfur colloid tend to be large, it is recommended that preparation should be slowly passed the dose through a 0.22-μ millipore filter before use.

Radiotracer injection can be given in many ways like intradermal, subdermal, subcutaneous, peritumoral, periareolar, and subareolar. For deep seated tumors, peritumoral injections, with or without ultrasound guidance, are advised. However, in most cases subdermal or intradermal injections are sufficient. If tumor is in the upper outer quadrant of breast, periareolar injection is recommended. Strong massage of the injection site is advised to support dose movement through lymphatics.

Injection is usually done on camera table, so that imaging can be done immediately. SLN can be seen within minutes. Images should be acquired every 5 min. SLNs are seen usually within 1 h. The location of the highest tracer activity on the skin was identified using a handheld gamma probe before taking incision (tracer activity should be at least two times higher than the background activity).

In a multicenter trial, Lorraine et al. included 529 patients who underwent SLNB procedure using a combination of blue dye and 99 m TC SC. They demonstrated that the identification rate increased and the false-negative rate decreased to 90% and 4.3%, respectively, if surgeon has already performed more than 30 cases [26].

99 m Tc SC has also been tried in a patient with local recurrence. Julian J. et al. could map 83% SLN successfully with 90% axillary lymph node biopsy in patient with chest wall recurrence. They concluded SLNB has acceptable identification and biopsy rates in women with an isolated chest wall recurrence. However, the sample size was small and more studies are required in this regard [27].

5.10 Positron Emission Mammography

The earlier we detect the tumor of the breast the better will be the prognosis. Detection of smaller lesions will not only decrease the morbidity of surgery and chemotherapies but also increase the event free and overall survival period. Due to low metabolic tumor volume; smaller, especially subcentimetric lesion, are more likely to be missed in the whole body (WB) PET/CT due to smoothing and its partial volume effects. Three-dimensional Positron Emission Mammography (PEM) is a dedicated scanner for breast imaging that has higher spatial resolution and improved sensitivity for smaller lesions. Data from previous studies appear to support this prediction [28–30]. The patient protocol is similar to whole-body PET scanning. After a minimum of 4 h of fasting, the radiotracer 18F-FDG is injected and images are acquired after 50–60 min. The patient lies prone so that breasts hang freely in the scanner table. The usual imaging time is 15–20 min. Reconstructed slice thickness may vary depending on the breast size.

Almost all initial studies have shown sensitivity as 85–87% for malignant breast lesions [31–33]. During evaluation of 18 malignant breast lesions Levine et al. demonstrated sensitivity, specificity, and overall diagnostic accuracy of PEM as 86%, 91%, and 89%, respectively [31].

Meta-analysis was done by Caldarella et al. to find diagnostic accuracy for evaluation of women with suspected breast lesions by PEM. The pooled sensitivity and specificity were 85% and 79%, respectively. Pooled sensitivity of PEM was found 86% for invasive carcinomas compared to 81% for carcinoma in situ [34].

PEM was compared with WB PET for primary lesion detection by Schilling et al. and Kalinyak et al. Significantly better sensitivity of PEM in comparison to WB PET was demonstrated by both of them (92.8% versus 67.9%; 92% versus 56%, respectively) [30, 35].

Similarly, in a study done on 45 females, Yamamoto et al. found higher sensitivity of PEM (66.7%) in comparison to WB PET (13.3%) for lesion size less than 1 cm. Interestingly, both of these modalities have shown comparable results for lesion size 1 cm and larger [29].

Irma et al. quantitatively analyzed PEM by PUVmax (maximum uptake value) and LTB (lesion to background) for baseline imaging and response assessment after neoadjuvant chemotherapy with considering their pathological subtypes. Both PUVmax and LTB showed a significant correlation with pathological subtypes. However, response to neoadjuvant chemotherapy could not be predicted in terms of breast cancer biomarkers [36].

Detection of subcentimetric lesions with their metabolic characteristics is a great milestone in the management of breast cancers. Early detection with prognostication is the need of time for the management toward improvement in morbidity and mortality. PEM has proven its potential role in this field.

References

1. Avril N, Dose J, Janicke F, et al. Metabolic characterization of breast tumours with positron emission tomography using 18F-fluorodeoxyglucose. J Clin Oncol. 1996;14:1848–57.
2. Avril N, Scheidhauer K, Kuhun W. Breast cancer. In: Helmut J, Wieler R, Coleman E, editors. PET in clinical oncology. New York: Springer; 2000. p. 355–72.
3. Barranger E, Grahek D, Antoine M, et al. Evaluation of fluorodeoxyglucose positron emission tomography in the detection of axillary lymph node metastases in patients with early-stage breast cancer. Ann Surg Oncol. 2003;10:622–7.
4. Cook G, Houston S, Rubens R, et al. Detection of bone metastases in breast cancer by 18F-FDG PET: differing metabolic activity in osteoblastic and osteolytic lesions. J Clin Oncol. 1998;16:3375–9.
5. Dose Schwarz J, Bader M, Jenicke L, et al. Early prediction of response to chemotherapy in metastatic breast cancer using sequential 18F-FDG PET. J Nucl Med. 2005;46:1144–50.
6. Even-Sapir E, Metser U, Flusser G, et al. Assessment of malignant skeletal disease: initial experience with 18F-fluoride PET/CT and comparison between 18F-fluoride PET and 18F-fluoride PET/CT. J Nucl Med. 2004;45:272–8.
7. Kumar R, Alavi A. Fluorodeoxyglucose-PET in the management of breast cancer. Radiol Clin N Am. 2004;6:1113–22.
8. Manohar K, Mittal BR, Bhoil A, et al. Role of 18F-FDG PET/CT in identifying distant metastatic disease missed by conventional imaging in patients with locally advanced breast cancer. Nucl Med Commun. 2013;34:557–61.
9. Nakai T, Okuyama C, Kubota T, et al. Pitfalls of FDG PET for the diagnosis of osteoblastic bone metastases in patients with breast cancer. Eur J Nucl Med Mol Imaging. 2005;32:1253–8.
10. Schirrmeister H, Kuhn T, Guhlmann A, et al. Fluorine-18 2-deoxy-2-fluoro-D-glucose PET in the preoperative staging of breast cancer: comparison with the standard staging procedures. Eur J Nucl Med. 2001;28:351–8.
11. Sohn YM, Hong IK, Han K. Role of [18F]fluorodeoxyglucose positron emission tomography-computed tomography, sonography, and sonographically guided fine-needle aspiration biopsy in the diagnosis of axillary lymph nodes in patients with breast cancer: comparison of diagnostic performance. J Ultrasound Med Jun. 2014;33:1013–21.
12. Smith IC, Welch AE, Hutcheon AW, et al. Positron emission tomography using [18F] fluorodeoxy-D-glucose to predict the pathologic response of breast cancer to primary chemotherapy. J Clin Oncol. 2000;18:1676–88.
13. Santiago JF, Gonen M, Yeung H, et al. A retrospective analysis of the impact of 18F-FDG PET scans on clinical management of 133 breast cancer patients. Q J Nucl Med Mol Imaging. 2006;50:61–7.
14. Siggelkow W, Rath W, Buell U, et al. FDG PET and tumour markers in the diagnosis of recurrent and metastatic breast cancer. Eur J Nucl Med Mol Imaging. 2004;31:S118–24.
15. Townsend DW. A combined PET/CT scanner: the choices. J Nucl Med. 2001;42:533–4.
16. Trampal C, Maldonado A, Sancho Cuesta F, et al. Role of the positron emission tomography (PET) in suspected tumor recurrence when there are increased serum tumor markers. Rev Esp Med Nucl. 2000;19:279–87.
17. Ugrinska A, Bombardieri E, Stokkel MP, et al. Circulating tumor markers and nuclear medicine imaging modalities: breast, prostate and ovarian cancer. Q J Nucl Med. 2002;46:88–104.
18. Van der Hoeven JJ, Hoekstra OS, Comans EF, et al. Determinations of diagnostic performance of 18F-fluoro-deoxyglucose positron emission tomography for axillary staging in breast cancer. Ann Surg. 2002;236:619–24.
19. Zangheri B, Messa C, Picchio M, et al. PET/CT and breast cancer. Eur J Nucl Med Mol Imaging. 2004;1:112–7.

20. Veronesi U, Paganelli G, Viale G, et al. Sentinel lymph node biopsy and axillary dissection in breast cancer: results in a large series. J Natl Cancer Inst. 1999;91:368–73.
21. Lyman GH, Giuliano AE, Somerfield MR, et al. American Society of Clinical Oncology guideline recommendations for sentinel lymph node biopsy in early-stage breast cancer, J Clin Oncol. 2005;23: 7703–7720.
22. Veronesi U, Paganelli G, Viale G, et al. A randomized comparison of sentinel-node biopsy with routine axillary dissection in breast cancer. N Engl J Med. 2003;349:546–53.
23. Krag D, Weaver D, Ashikaga T, et al. The sentinel node in breast cancer a multicenter validation study. N Engl J Med. 1998;339:941–6.
24. Dauway EL, Giuliano R, Haddad F, et al. Lymphatic mapping in breast cancer. Hematol Oncol Clin North Am. 1999;13:349–71.
25. Margenthaler JA. Axillary sentinel lymph node biopsy. Philadelphia: Lippincott Williams & Wilkins; 2011.
26. Lorraine T, Donald R, Melvin S, et al. Multicenter trial of sentinel node biopsy for breast cancer using both technetium sulfur colloid and Isosulfan blue dye. Ann Surg. 2001;233(1):51–9.
27. Julian J, Laura E, Cheryl E, et al. Sentinel lymph node mapping in post-mastectomy Chest Wall recurrences: influence on radiation treatment fields and outcome. Ann Surg Oncol. 2016;23:715–21.
28. Thompson CJ, Murthy K, Weinbera IN, Mako F. Feasibility study for positron emission mammography. Med Phys. 1994;21(4):529–38.
29. Y. Yamamoto, Y. Ozawa, K. Kubouchi, S. Nakamura, Y. Nakajima, and T. Inoue, Comparative analysis of imaging sensitivity of positron emission mammography and whole-body PET in relation to tumor size," Clin Nucl Med, vol. 40, no. 1, pp. 21–25, 2015.
30. Schilling K, Narayanan D, Kalinyak JE, et al. Positron emission mammography in breast cancer presurgical planning: comparisons with magnetic resonance imaging. Eur J Nucl Med Mol Imaging. 2011;38(1):23–36.
31. Levine EA, Freimanis RI, Perrier ND, et al. Positron emission mammography: initial clinical results. Ann Surg Oncol. 2003;10:86–91.
32. Rosen EL, Turkington TG, Soo MS, Baker JA, Coleman RE. Detection of primary breast carcinoma with a dedicated, large-field-of-view FDG PET mammography device: initial experience. Radiology. 2005;234(2):527–34.
33. Tafra L, Cheng Z, Uddo J, et al. Pilot clinical trial of FDG positron emission mammography in the surgical management of breast cancer. Ann Surg Oncol. 2005;190:628–32.
34. Caldarella C, Treglia G, Giordano A. Diagnostic performance of dedicated positron emission mammography using fluorine-18-fluorodeoxyglucose in women with suspicious breast lesions: a meta-analysis. Clin Breast Cancer. 2014;14(4):241–8.
35. Kalinyak JE, Berg WA, Schilling K, et al. Breast cancer detection using high-resolution breast WBPET compared to whole-body WBPET or WBPET/CT. Eur J Nucl Med Mol Imaging. 2014;41:260–75.
36. Irma S, Sevastian S, Cynthia V, et al. Usefulness of positron emission mammography in the evaluation of response to neoadjuvant chemotherapy in patients with breast cancer. Am J Nucl Med Mol Imaging. 2018;8(5):341–50.

FDG-PET/CT in Breast Cancer: Normal Variants, Artifacts, and Pitfalls

6

Ameya D. Puranik and Ashmi S. Manglunia

Contents

6.1 Introduction

PET/CT has a crucial role in the evaluation of locally advanced or metastatic breast cancer. However, to appropriately interpret an FDG-PET/CT study, it is essential to be familiar with the normal physiologic distribution of FDG uptake and to recognize various physiologic variants, artifacts, and potential pitfalls.

As an imaging tool for breast cancer, PET/CT has a few shortcomings despite having many advantages. A variable sensitivity (range 63%–96%) and specificity (range 75%–100%) of PET/CT in evaluating primary breast lesions has been reported in the literature [1–4]. It is important to understand the spectrum of benign breast processes, be familiar with their pattern of FDG uptake and accompanying CT findings. In this chapter, discuss the various artifacts and pitfalls of benign lesions that should be recognized in evaluation of breast cancer.

A. D. Puranik (✉)
Department of Nuclear Medicine and Molecular Imaging, Tata Memorial Hospital, Parel, Mumbai, India

Homi Bhabha National Institute, Mumbai, India

A. S. Manglunia
Molecular Imaging and Therapy, Delhi, India

59

6.1.1 Normal Variants

6.1.1.1 Physiological Breast Changes

Dense Breasts
Dense breasts exhibit, on average, higher FDG uptake than non-dense breasts [5]. This increased uptake is usually symmetric, bilateral, and diffuse, with no lesion seen on the corresponding CT. However, uptake in dense breasts may mask small and low-grade tumors causing false-negative results.

Menstrual Cycle
Lin et al. [6] observed a significant correlation between the FDG uptake in breast and the menstrual cycle. They postulated that FDG studies are less sensitive in detecting small breast tumors during the ovulatory and secretory phases.

Lactation
Lactating breasts may also show increased diffuse FDG uptake as a result of increased expression of the insulin-independent glucose transporter, GLUT-1, and absence of the insulin-dependent transporter, GLUT-4, in the lactating breast [7].

Gynaecomastia
The most common cause of male breast enlargement, and can be unilateral. Histologic pattern associated with gynecomastia is the proliferation of stroma and ducts. This may show unilateral increased tracer uptake in the breast.

6.1.1.2 Iatrogenic Changes

Silicone Granulomata
Focal FDG uptake can be seen in the augmented or reconstructed breast, post-silicone augmentation. Silicone causes an inflammatory reaction in the soft tissues and thus, it is not uncommon for intense FDG uptake to be observed in the ipsilateral axillary lymph nodes of a patient with ruptured breast implants [8].

Fat Necrosis
Common causes include surgery, radiation therapy, and trauma. Fat necrosis is a sterile inflammatory process that results in increased uptake due to the presence of inflammatory cells [9]. A history of trauma, prior surgery, and mammographic finding of characteristic oil cysts and calcifications is helpful for diagnosis.

Hematoma
Hematomas can occur following trauma, biopsy, or surgery. Associated inflammatory reactions and granulation tissue can show increased FDG uptake. However, as the hematoma evolves, the uptake subsides.

Post-surgery/Radiotherapy

Increased FDG uptake may be observed in the postoperative period (Fig. 6.1) due to leukocyte infiltration at the site of wound repair and resorption of necrotic debris. Similar increased uptake is seen in post-radiotherapy due to inflammation at the site of normal structures.

This abnormal uptake may mimic residual disease or mask malignant FDG uptake in neighboring structures. It is, thus, advisable to schedule a PET/CT study at least 6 weeks post-surgery or radiotherapy. Dual time-point FDG-PET has also been suggested to allow for better differentiation between cancer and inflammatory changes, although controversial. Further, post-operative seromas are commonly seen which are well-defined serous fluid collections in the chest wall with minimal or absent FDG uptake (Fig. 6.2).

Node Uptake Due to Infiltration

Extravasation of radiotracer at the injection site can result in subcutaneous tracking of FDG along lymphatics in the arm, resulting in axillary node uptake. Injection at the side contralateral to the site of disease is advised to differentiate between artifactual and metastatic uptake. In case the injection is on the side of primary malignancy, CT features of the nodes (fatty hilum, shape, etc.) can be used to differentiate between reactive/metastatic pattern, though not a foolproof method.

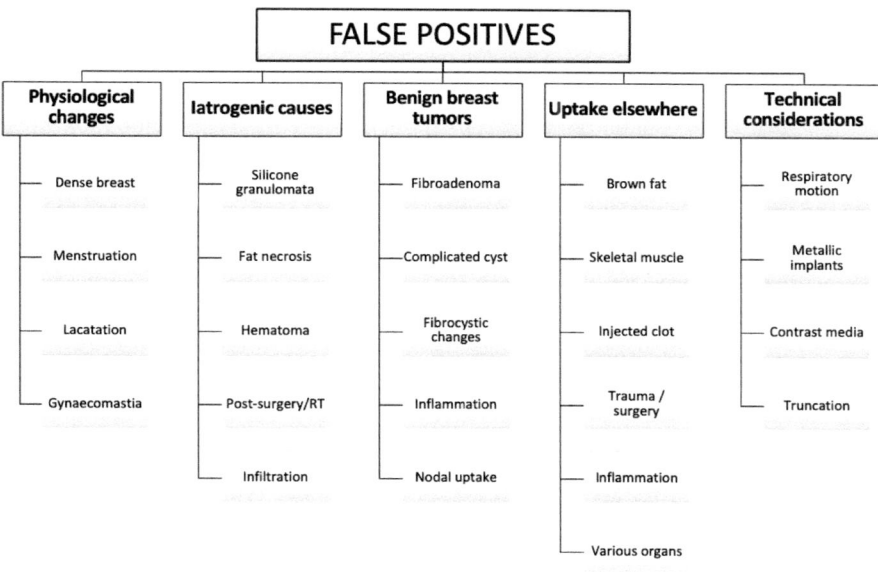

Fig. 6.1 False positives on PET/CT imaging

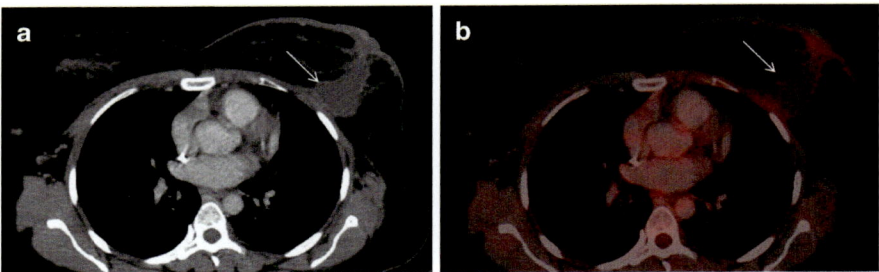

Fig. 6.2 Patient is a 62-year-old lady, operated case of carcinoma left breast, FDG-PET/CT scan for done for evaluation of disease status, since patient complained of sudden weight loss. Axial CT (**a**) and fused PET/CT (**b**) images show a well-defined cystic lesion (arrow in **a**) overlying the pectoral muscles with patchy areas of low-grade FDG uptake (arrow in **b**)—represents a post-operative seroma

6.1.2 Benign Breast Tumors

Fibroadenomas
Fibroadenomas are one of the most common benign tumors of the breast. Mild focal FDG uptake can be seen within the fibroadenoma as a consequence of their high proliferation (Fig. 6.3), more often noted in complex fibroadenomas. Complex fibroadenomas can mimic malignancy (Fig. 6.4) by their propensity to show increased uptake along with increasing size [10].

Complicated Cysts
Complicated cysts contain proteinaceous fluid, cholesterol crystal, blood, or other material, which can cause inflammation in the cyst wall and result in FDG uptake. A complicated cyst can present on CT as a fluid-filled breast mass with homogeneous rim enhancement.

Fibrocystic Changes
Fibrocystic breast disease, also referred to as fibrocystic change, affects more than 60% of women. FDG uptake related to fibrocystic change tends to be diffuse.

Inflammation
FDG uptake is seen at sites of infection or inflammation due to the associated leukocytic infiltration. The cause is usually mastitis or rarely, an abscess. In a few such cases, inflammatory breast cancer needs to be excluded. Alberini and colleagues [11] showed that PET/CT scan was positive for inflammatory breast cancer in 100% and false positive in 2 of 3 patients with benign mastitis.

Diabetic mastopathy of the breast is another uncommon tumor-like fibrous proliferation of the breast seen mostly in premenopausal women with type I diabetes mellitus and can be FDG avid. A core biopsy is usually recommended for diagnosis [12].

Fig. 6.3 In a patient with suspected breast neoplasm, FDG-PET/CT was done after equivocal mammographic findings. Axial CT (**a**) and fused PET/CT (**b**) images show a well-defined solid-density lesion in left breast (arrow in **a**) with no significant FDG uptake (arrow in **b**) suggestive of a fibroadenoma

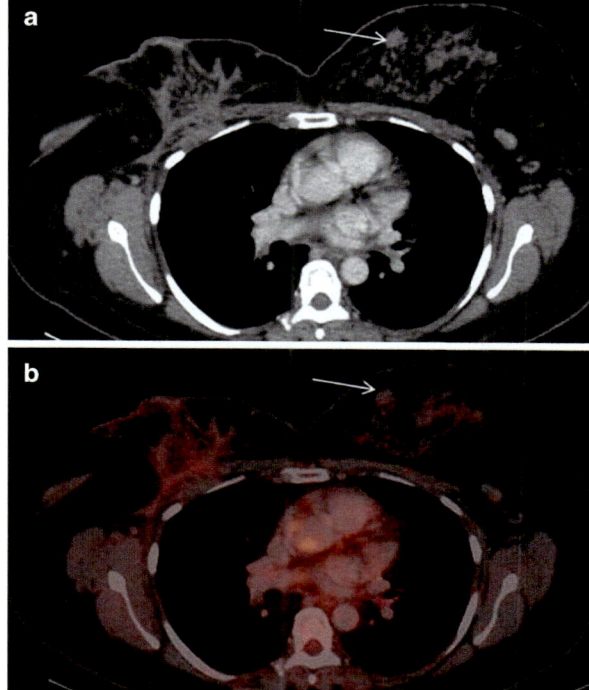

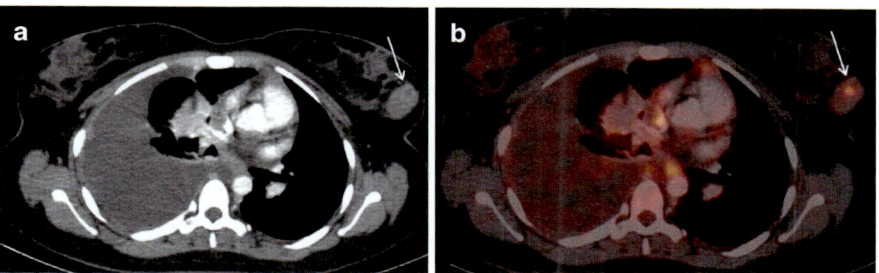

Fig. 6.4 In a 52-year-old lady with palpable left breast lump, Axial CT (**a**) and fused FDG-PET/CT (**b**) images show FDG-avid enhancing lesion in left breast (arrows), which on histopathological analysis reveal complex fibroadenoma

Nodal Uptake

FDG uptake can be seen in benign axillary lymph nodes following immunization [13], inflammatory conditions [14] or from adjacent mastitis.

One also has to keep in mind the possibility of a FDG-avid lesion in breast to be a metastatic deposit from a primary neoplasm somewhere else in the body. Other malignancies, like lymphoma, can also mimic a primary breast malignancy.

6.1.3   Artifacts and Pitfalls

6.1.3.1 Elsewhere in the Body in Breast Cancer Assessment
Brown fat
The tracer uptake in brown adipose tissue is well recognized and occurs frequently in patients with low body mass index and in cold weather (Fig. 6.5). Glucose accumulation within brown fat is increased by sympathetic stimulation and can be identified easily due to its characteristic distribution.

Skeletal Muscle Uptake
Physiologic muscle uptake is commonly encountered in studies due to excessive muscle activity during the uptake phase or within a few days preceding the study. Insulin or recent food intake can also give rise to the same. To avoid this, patients should rest comfortably during the uptake phase. Muscle relaxants such as benzodiazepines may also be used [15].

Injected Clot
At the time of radiotracer administration, blood withdrawal in syringe can lead to injection of radioactive clot, resulting in pulmonary hotspots. The absence of a CT correlate for a pulmonary hotspot should raise the possibility of the injected clot.

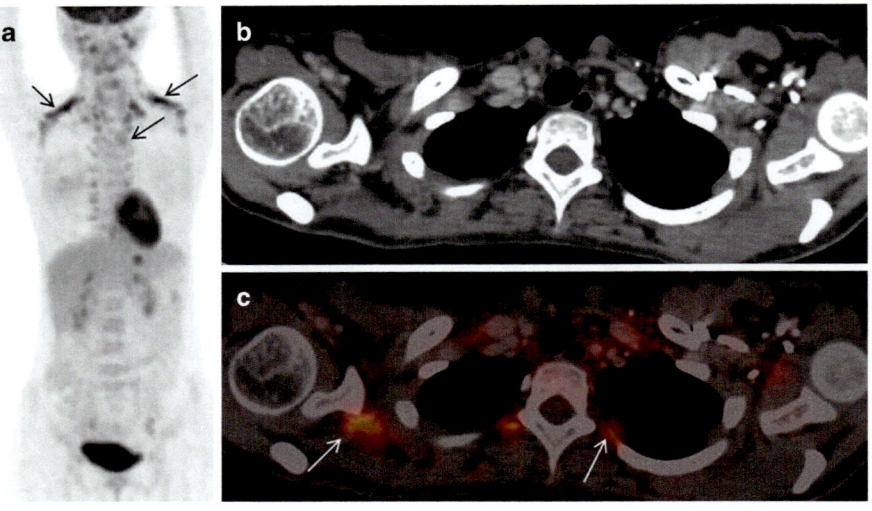

Fig. 6.5 Symmetrically increased FDG uptake in bilateral lower neck and midline abdominal regions on MIP image (**a**—arrows), which corresponds to FDG uptake in bilateral supraclavicular and intercostal region in region of fat seen on axial PET/CT (**b**) and CT (**c**) images, respectively—suggestive of brown adipose tissue

Trauma or Surgery

Osseous injury from traumatic or iatrogenic causes can lead to increased tracer uptake on PET due to accumulation of inflammatory cells during the active repair and healing process.

Thymic Hyperplasia

Increased FDG uptake in the anterior mediastinum can be attributed to thymic hyperplasia by identification of a triangular soft tissue density seen retrosternally on CT. Prominent thymic uptake may also be seen following chemotherapy.

Uterine Uptake

The endometrium of premenopausal females usually shows cyclically variable uptake, with marked uptake seen during menstruation [16]. Marked uptake is also associated with fibroid tumors in some cases [16]. Endometrial uptake in postmenopausal women is usually abnormal and warrants further investigation.

Ovarian Uptake

Inflammatory processes, ovulating ovaries, and corpus luteum cysts may cause focal increased uptake [17].

Marrow Uptake

Increased homogenous FDG uptake is commonly observed in the marrow and spleen following GCSF therapy; usually resolving within 1 month. It is advisable to postpone FDG-PET until approximately 4 weeks after treatment. Increased diffuse uptake can also be seen with hyperplasia and hematopoietic stimulation from anemia.

Reduced bone marrow FDG uptake can be noted several months after radiation therapy, attributed to the replacement of bone marrow by fatty tissue [18].

Infection/Inflammation

Focal increased FDG accumulation is seen with various infectious or inflammatory processes such as abscesses, pneumonia, osteomyelitis, tuberculosis, and fungal or granulomatous disease.

6.1.3.2 Technical Artifacts

Respiratory Motion

PET is acquired over several breathing cycles while CT, over a single phase of the breathing cycle. This introduces a mismatch between the CT attenuation data and the PET emission data. A rib lesion could potentially overlap breast tissue, simulating FDG-avid breast malignancy. Additionally, this type of artifact can have an impact on patients with liver lesions [19].

Metallic Implants

Metallic implants such as dental fillings, prosthetics, or chemotherapy ports result in high CT numbers and generate streaking artifacts. This results in correspondingly high PET attenuation coefficients, leading to a false-positive PET finding. Similar false-positive findings can be seen in breast implants too. Comparison of the attenuation corrected and the non-attenuation-corrected images aids in avoiding misinterpretation.

Contrast Media

High-contrast concentrations result in high CT numbers because of photon absorption [20], leading to an overestimation of tracer uptake. Artifacts representing intense focal accumulations of positive oral contrast material can usually be resolved by viewing the CT and non-attenuation-corrected PET scans. The use of negative-attenuation oral contrast also serves to resolve the problem.

Truncation

Truncation artifacts in PET/CT are due to the size difference in the field of view between the CT (50 cm) and PET (70 cm) tomographs [21]. Large patients will have PET data without corresponding CT attenuation factors and resulting in underestimated SUVs. Careful patient positioning is crucial to reduce these artifacts.

6.1.4   False Negatives

Small Tumor Size

PET has limited sensitivity in detecting lesions less than 10 mm. PET/CT also may not detect a lesion beyond the resolution of CT, which is about 4 mm. Also, recent studies have shown that SUV decreases as the size of the lesion decreases, which can contribute to higher false-negative rates [4].

Histologic Tumor Type and Tumor Grade

False-negative results are reported in slow-growing and well-differentiated histologic subtypes of tumors such as tubular carcinoma, in situ carcinoma, and lobular carcinoma [22, 23].

Tissue Heterogeneity

Malignant cells contribute from a few to more than 90% of the tumor, whereas up to 10% is contributed by inflammatory cells and non-metabolically active components, that is, necrotic tissue, fibrotic scar, or mucin. Therefore, minimal FDG uptake by these cells can affect the overall results of PET imaging.

Blood Glucose Levels

FDG uptake by cancer cells tends to decline as blood glucose and insulin levels increase. Wahl and colleagues [24] showed that increasing levels of glucose lead to inhibition of FDG uptake in breast cancer cells. Thus, FDG-PET imaging in uncontrolled diabetic patients may lead to false-negative results.

Brain Lesions

FDG-PET has limited application in detecting skull and brain metastases because of high uptake by normal cerebral gray matter.

Accurate PET-CT interpretation requires awareness of the pitfalls associated with the imaging components, to avoid misdiagnosis, overstaging of disease, and unnecessary biopsies.

References

1. Adler LP, Crowe JP, Al-Kaisi NK, Sunshine JL. Evaluation of breast masses and axillary lymph nodes with [F-18] 2-deoxy-2-fluoro-D-glucose PET. Radiology. 1993;187(3): 743–50.
2. Kumar R, Chauhan A, Zhuang H, Chandra P, Schnall M, Alavi A. Clinicopathologic factors associated with false negative FDG–PET in primary breast cancer. Breast Cancer Res Treat. 2006;98(3):267–74.
3. Avril N, Rosé CA, Schelling M, Dose J, Kuhn W, Bense S, et al. Breast imaging with positron emission tomography and fluorine-18 fluorodeoxyglucose: use and limitations. J Clin Oncol. 2000;18:3495–502.
4. Kumar R, Loving VA, Chauhan A, Zhuang H, Mitchell S, Alavi A. Potential of dual-time-point imaging to improve breast cancer diagnosis with (18)F-FDG PET. J Nucl Med. 2005;46(11):1819–24.
5. Vranjesevic D, Schiepers C, Silverman DH, Quon A, Villalpando J, Dahlbom M, et al. Relationship between 18F-FDG uptake and breast density in women with normal breast tissue. J Nucl Med. 2003;44(8):1238–42.
6. Lin CY, Ding HJ, Liu CS, Chen YK, Lin CC, Kao CH. Correlation between the intensity of breast FDG uptake and menstrual cycle. Acad Radiol. 2007;14(8):940–4.
7. Hicks RJ, Binns D, Stabin MG. Pattern of uptake and excretion of (18) F-FDG in the lactating breast. J Nucl Med. 2001;42(8):1238–42.
8. Hurwitz R. F-18 FDG positron emission tomographic imaging in a case of ruptured breast implant: inflammation or recurrent tumor? Clin Nucl Med. 2003;28(9):755–6.
9. Tan PH, Lai LM, Carrington EV, Opaluwa AS, Ravikumar KH, Chetty N, et al. Fat necrosis of the breast: a review. Breast. 2006;15(3):313–8.
10. Makis W, Ciarallo A, Hickeson M, Derbekyan V. Rapidly growing complex fibroadenoma with surrounding ductal hyperplasia mimics breast malignancy on serial F-18 FDG PET/CT imaging. Clin Nucl Med. 2011;36(7):576–9.
11. Alberini JL, Lerebours F, Wartski M, Fourme E, Le Stanc E, Gontier E, et al. 18F-fluorodeoxyglucose positron emission tomography/ computed tomography (FDG-PET/CT) imaging in the staging and prognosis of inflammatory breast cancer. Cancer. 2009;115(21):5038–47.
12. Baratelli GM, Riva C. Diabetic fibrous mastopathy: sonographic-pathologic correlation. J Clin Ultrasound. 2005;33(1):34–7.
13. Williams G, Joyce RM, Parker JA. False-positive axillary lymph node on FDG-PET/CT scan resulting from immunization. Clin Nucl Med. 2006;31(11):731–2.
14. Prosch H, Mirzaei S, Oschatz E, Strasser G, Huber M, Mostbeck G. Case report: gluteal injection site granulomas: false positive finding on FDG-PET in patients with non-small cell lung cancer. Br J Radiol. 2005;78(932):758–61.
15. Yeung HW, Grewal RK, Gonen M, Schoder H, Larson SM. Patterns of (18)F-FDG uptake in adipose tissue and muscle: a potential source of false-positives for PET. J Nucl Med. 2003;44(11):1789–96.
16. Subhas N, Patel PV, Pannu HK, Jacene HA, Fishman EK, Wahl RL. Imaging of pelvic malignancies with in-line FDG PET-CT: case examples and common pitfalls of FDG PET. Radiographics. 2005;25(4):1031–43.

17. Lerman H, Metser U, Grisaru D, Fishman A, Lievshitz G, Even-Sapir E. Normal and abnormal 18F-FDG endometrial and ovarian uptake in pre- and postmenopausal patients: assessment by PET/ CT. J Nucl Med. 2004;45(2):266–71.
18. Alavi A, Gupta N, Alberini JL, Hickeson M, Adam LE, Bhargava P, et al. Positron emission tomography imaging in nonmalignant thoracic disorders. Semin Nucl Med. 2002;32(4):293–321.
19. Osman MM, Cohade C, Nakamoto Y, Wahl RL. Respiratory motion artifacts on PET emission images obtained using CT attenuation correction on PET-CT. Eur J Nucl Med Mol Imaging. 2003;30:603–6.
20. Cohade C, Osman M, Nakamoto Y, Marshall LT, Links JM, Fishman EK, et al. Initial experience with oral contrast in PET/CT: phantom and clinical studies. J Nucl Med. 2003;44(3):412–6.
21. Mawlawi O, Pan T, Cody DD, et al. Evaluation of a new CT truncation correction algorithm for accurate quantification of PET/CT images. J Nucl Med. 2004;45(suppl):413P.
22. Avril N, Menzel M, Dose J, Schelling M, Weber W, Jänicke F, et al. Glucose metabolism of breast cancer assessed by ^{18}F-FDG PET: histologic and immunohistochemical tissue analysis. J Nucl Med. 2001;42(1):9–16.
23. Buck A, Schirrmeister H, Kuhn T, Shen C, Kalker T, Kotzerke J, et al. FDG uptake in breast cancer: correlation with biological and clinical prognostic parameters. Eur J Nucl Med Mol Imaging. 2002;29(10):1317–23.
24. Wahl RL, Cody RL, Hutchins GD, Mudgett EE. Primary and metastatic breast carcinoma: initial clinical evaluation with PET with the radiolabeled glucose analogue 2-[F-18]-fluoro-2-deoxy-D-glucose. Radiology. 1991;179(3):765–70.

Recent Advances in Molecular Imaging of Breast Cancer

7

P. Sai Sradha Patro, Girish Kumar Parida, and Kanhaiyalal Agrawal

Contents

7.1   Novel Tracers Used in Management of Breast Carcinoma

With time breast cancer treatments are becoming more and more precise with the aim to target specific pathways of tumorigenesis. Accordingly, more sophisticated imaging modalities are coming up for more accurate diagnosis, response assessment, and prognosis. 18F-FDG PET-CT has been an important milestone in this path. However, due to the lack of specificity of 18F-FDG for detection of selective targets, and malignancies, many novel PET biomarkers have been investigated (Table 7.1) [1–5]. Among others, estrogen receptor-based and human epidermal growth factor receptor 2 (HER2)-based imaging are of significant value as they are specific to breast cancer. Besides, a few other tracers specific for cancer have also been tried as diagnostic as well as theragnostic purposes.

P. S. S. Patro · G. K. Parida · K. Agrawal (✉)
Department of Nuclear Medicine, All India Institute of Medical Sciences, Bhubaneswar, India

© The Author(s), under exclusive license to Springer Nature Switzerland AG 2023
R. Kumar et al. (eds.), *PET/CT in Breast Cancer*, Clinicians' Guides to Radionuclide Hybrid Imaging, https://doi.org/10.1007/978-3-031-29590-4_7

Table 7.1 Various novel PET tracers under research for breast cancer

New tracers	Target receptor/mechanism of uptake	Useful for
^{18}F-FES	Estrogen receptor	Response to hormonal therapy, prognostication
89Zr-DFO-trastuzumab/68Ga-F(ab′)2- trastuzumab	HER 2/neu expression	Prognostication, Trastuzumab treatment option, and response evaluation
^{18}F-FDHT	Androgen receptor expression	New targeted therapy option for MBC
^{18}F-FTT	PARP-1 inhibitor	Targeted therapy inhibiting DNA repair
^{18}F-FLT	Thymidine kinase activity	Proliferation marker for therapy response
^{18}F-FMISO	Hypoxia (tumor environment)	Prognostication (predicts therapy response)
[18]F-annexin V	Apoptosis (phosphatidylserine expression on cell)	Biomarker for drug resistance
[11]C-MET/^{18}F-FET	Amino acid metabolism	Staging and response evaluation
[11]C-Choline/^{18}F-Flurocholine	Membrane synthesis of cells	Proliferation marker, useful to detect leptomeningeal spread
[11]C/^{18}F-PgP targeted tracers	Breast cancer-resistant protein	Drug resistance analysis
[18]F/^{68}Ga-RGD derivatives	$\alpha_v\beta_3$ Integrins	Antiangiogenic therapy monitoring
^{68}Ga-DOTAGA-IAC	$\alpha_v\beta_3$ Integrin antagonist	Antiangiogenic therapy monitoring
[89]Zr-Atezolizumab	PD-L1	Targeted immunotherapy in MBC
[89]Zr-Bevacizumab	VEGF	For antiangiogenic therapy
^{68}Ga-RM2(Bombesin)	Gastrin releasing peptide receptor antagonist	Noninvasive evaluation of ER-positive status in MBC
^{68}Ga-FAPI-04/46	Fibroblast activated protein	Initial diagnosis, staging, and response evaluation
^{68}Ga-PSMA-11	Tumor neovascularization	Possible radioligand therapy option
[68]Ga-Pentixafor	CXCR4-ligand (chemokine receptor)	Initial, recurrent evaluation, and for targeted therapy in invasive breast cancer
[64]Cu-DOTA-alendronate	Mammary microcalcifications	Differentiation of malignant versus benign breast tumors
[64]Cu-M5A	Anti-carcinoembryonic antigen (CEA) antibody	CEA positivity status (prognostication)

FES 16α-18F-fluoro-17β-estradiol, *FDHT* fluorodihydrotesterone, *MBC* metastatic breast cancer, *FTT* fluorothanatrace, *PARP* poly ADP ribose polymerase, *FLT* fluorothymidine, *FMISO* fluoromisonidazole, *MET* methionine, *FET* fluoroethyltyrosine, *PgP* P glycoprotein, *RGD* arginine-glycine-aspartame, *FAPI* fibroblast-activation protein inhibitors, *PSMA* prostate-specific membrane antigen, *M5A* monoclonal antibody, *PD-L1* programmed death-ligand 1, *VEGF* vascular endothelial growth factor

7.1.1 Estrogen Receptor Imaging

Every three out of four patients with breast cancer usually express estrogen receptor (ER) [6]. It is important to know the ER expression status of the tumor in such patients, as ER-positive tumors respond well to the anti-hormonal therapy whereas ER-negative tumors usually do not respond to them [7]. In general, the assessment of ER status of the tumor is performed by immunohistochemistry (IHC) of the biopsy specimen of the primary tumor. Although IHC is considered as gold standard, studies have revealed that it can predict response to hormonal therapy in only about half of the patients [8]. A few factors that affect the result include interobserver variation and delay-to-fixation time [9]. Besides these, recent studies showed that in approximately 20% of cases worldwide the IHC results may be inaccurate due to tumor heterogeneity [10].

Whole-body PET with 16α-18F-fluoro-17β-estradiol (18F-FES) is a unique noninvasive modality for obtaining about the ER expression in the lesions [11]. Literature evidence shows that 18F-FES PET is capable of detecting ER receptor status of the tumor and the intensity of tracer uptake has a good correlation with the IHC scoring [12, 13]. A meta-analysis has reported pooled sensitivity and specificity of 18F-FES PET to be 82% and 95%, respectively, for detecting ER-positive tumor lesions in breast cancer [14].

Besides being noninvasive, there are a few other advantages of 18F FES PET over the conventional IHC results. In case of recurrent disease, re-biopsy is considered to be the gold standard. However, sometimes due to the location of lesion or associated comorbidities, re-biopsy of lesion is less feasible, and noninvasive 18F FES PET can be used in such scenarios. Importantly, the ER receptor expression within a patient across different metastatic lesions or within a tumor itself, may not be similar and can be heterogeneous. Further, a single-site biopsy in such a patient may not be representative of the overall ER expression and can lead to sampling bias. A noninvasive method like 18F FES PET would therefore be greatly beneficial for quantifying ER expression in such situations. A prospective cohort study has reported a good correlation between 18F FES PET-CT positivity and IHC status with a positive and negative predictive values of 100% and 78%, respectively [15]. Various trials on clinical utility of 18F FES PET-CT in response evaluation to hormonal therapy are ongoing. The outcome of these trials will impact the further widespread use of 18F FES PET-CT in breast cancer imaging.

7.1.2 HER2 Targeted Imaging

Breast carcinoma with HER2 overexpression has been proven to be aggressive in nature, and its expression not only can prognosticate but also is capable of directly influencing the management. Therefore, HER2 receptor has become an important target for imaging as well as therapy [16, 17]. About 20% of breast cancer patients usually overexpress HER2. These patients can get significant benefits from the HER2 targeted therapies [18]. Besides, HER2-positive tumors, it has also been seen that approximately 10% of patients with primary HER2-negative tumors have also shown clinical benefits to HER2 targeted therapy [19]. This is due to the heterogeneity of receptor expression not just in primary tumors, but in metastatic diseases as well [20]. HER2 targeted imaging, with PET and SPECT tracers can assess the heterogeneity and discrepancy between primary as well as metastatic diseases. A few commonly used tracers for HER2 PET imaging include 89Zr-DFO-trastuzumab, 64Cu-DOTA-trastuzumab, and 68Ga-F(ab')2- trastuzumab. These PET imaging methods have been used as noninvasive tools to evaluate HER2-positive primary and metastatic lesions. Radiolabeled antibodies, antibody fragments, and affibody molecules enable PET imaging to be a reliable and quantitative method for detecting HER2-positive cancer [21]. Both ER and HER2-targeted PET imaging have the potential to be useful noninvasive tools in the routine clinical care of patients with breast cancer.

7.1.3 Proliferation Marker

Anticancer therapeutic drugs targeting tumor proliferation have been used for metastatic breast cancer. Imaging with proliferation markers can be useful for initial staging, response evaluation, and follow-up of patients being treated with these drugs. 3'-deoxy-3'-[18 F] fluorothymidine (18FLT) is a PET imaging biomarker for in vivo imaging of cell proliferation. It is retained in the proliferating cells via thymidine kinase-1. Furthermore, it strongly correlates with the immuno-histological proliferation index Ki-67 [22]. 18FLT PET-CT has been found useful to prognosticate and predict early response to various chemotherapeutic drugs [23]. Hence, it can be useful in identifying treatment responders early after initiating a chemotherapeutic regimen in metastatic breast cancer which can impact further management.

7.1.4 Hypoxia Imaging

Hypoxic microenvironment developed due to excess growth of tumor cells facilitates its metastatic spread, resistance to apoptosis, hence results in poor response to therapy via various genetic and metabolic adaptive processes. Thus, acts as a poor prognostic factor affecting the overall survival of breast cancer as well [24]. Noninvasive ways of assessing tumor microenvironment will be useful in prognosticating and planning management in breast cancer. 18F-fluoromisonidazole (18F-MISO) PET demonstrates tumor hypoxia noninvasively in various cancers. Its utility in breast cancer needs to be further explored by multicenter studies.

7.1.5 Angiogenesis Imaging

Integrin αvβ3 has been found to be upregulated in the tumor neo-vasculature and is involved in tumor transformation, angiogenesis, local invasiveness, and metastatic potential. Hence found to be an important prognostication marker predicting survival in metastatic breast cancer. ^{18}F/^{68}Ga-arginine-glycine-aspartic acid (RGD) peptide derivative PET-CT tracers have been found useful in mapping tumor angiogenesis noninvasively both in primary and in metastatic lesions in breast cancer (Figs. 7.1, 7.2, and 7.3). This guides in treatment planning with antiangiogenetic molecules and monitoring its response [25]. It has to be further validated with large-scale studies for routine clinical use.

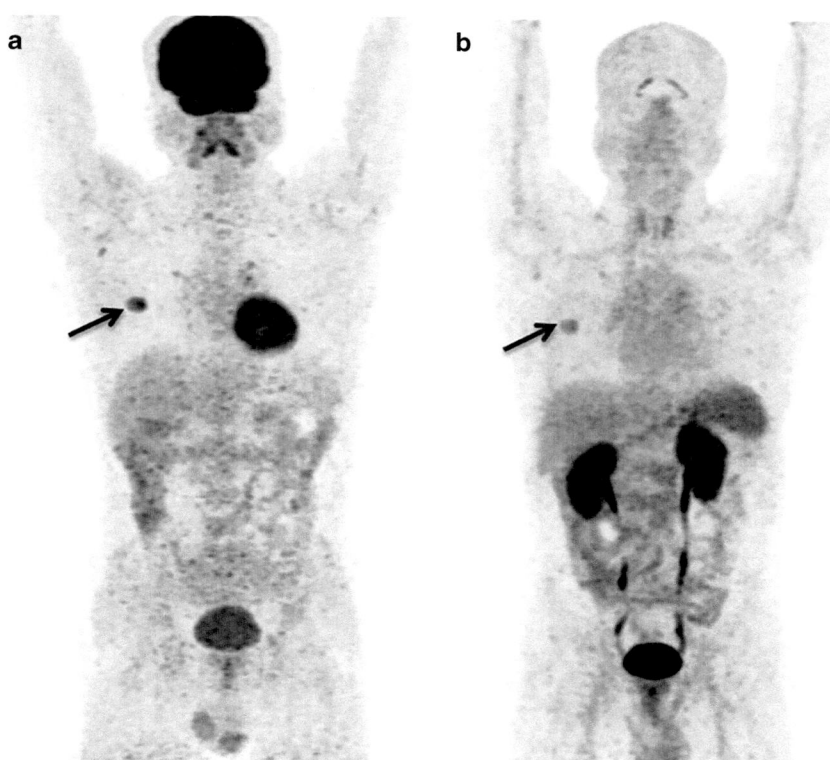

Fig. 7.1 A 52-year-old male with right breast invasive ductal carcinoma, clinical stage T4b N1 M0. Maximum intensity projection (MIP) 18F-FDG PET image demonstrates tracer uptake in the right thoracic region with SUVmax 9.7 (arrow in **a**). MIP 68Ga-DOTAGA-IAC PET image demonstrates the integrin receptor expression in the same lesion with SUVmax 3.71 (arrow in **b**)

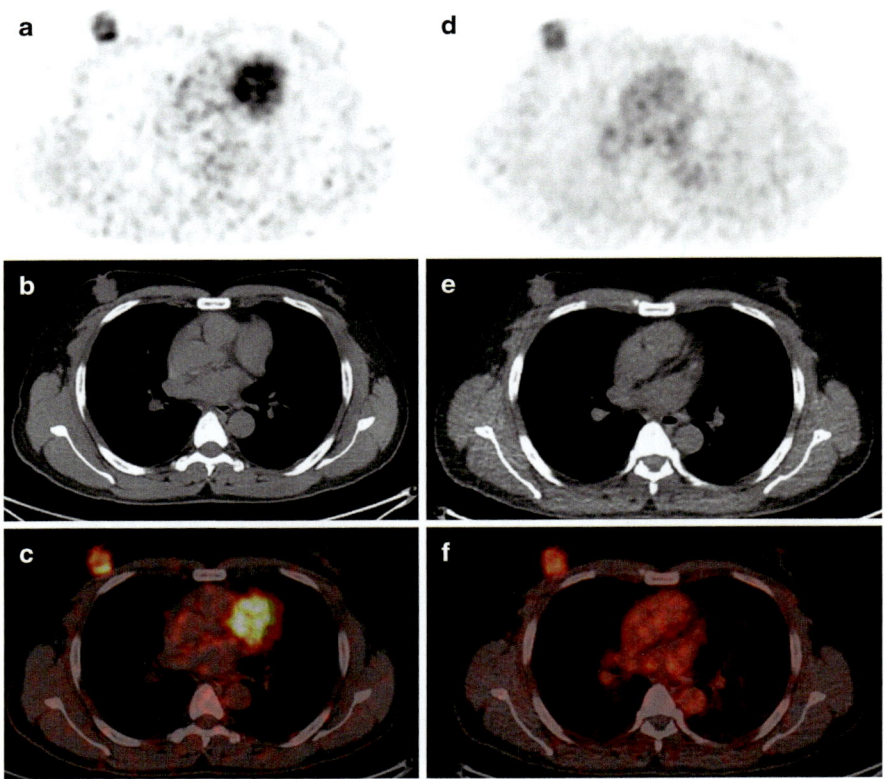

Fig. 7.2 Axial 18F-FDG PET/CT images (**a–c**) show tracer avid right retroareolar soft tissue lesion with SUVmax 9.7. Axial 68Ga-DOTAGA-IAC PET/CT images (**d–f**) show tracer avidity in the same lesion with SUVmax 3.71

7.1.6   Tumor Neovascularization Imaging

68Ga-Prostate specific membrane antigen (PSMA)-11 PET-CT targets the PSMA overexpression in tumor neovascularization. It was found to be overexpressed in invasive ductal carcinoma, triple-negative breast cancer, and signet cell adenocarcinoma of breast. Hence 68Ga PSMA PET-CT can play a complementary role in low FDG avid breast cancer and can also be explored for its theranaostic role in selecting patients with progressive metastatic breast cancer for targeted radioligand therapy, like with 177Lu-PSMA/225-Ac-PSMA-617 [26]. Further studies are needed to validate its theragnostic role in metastatic breast cancer.

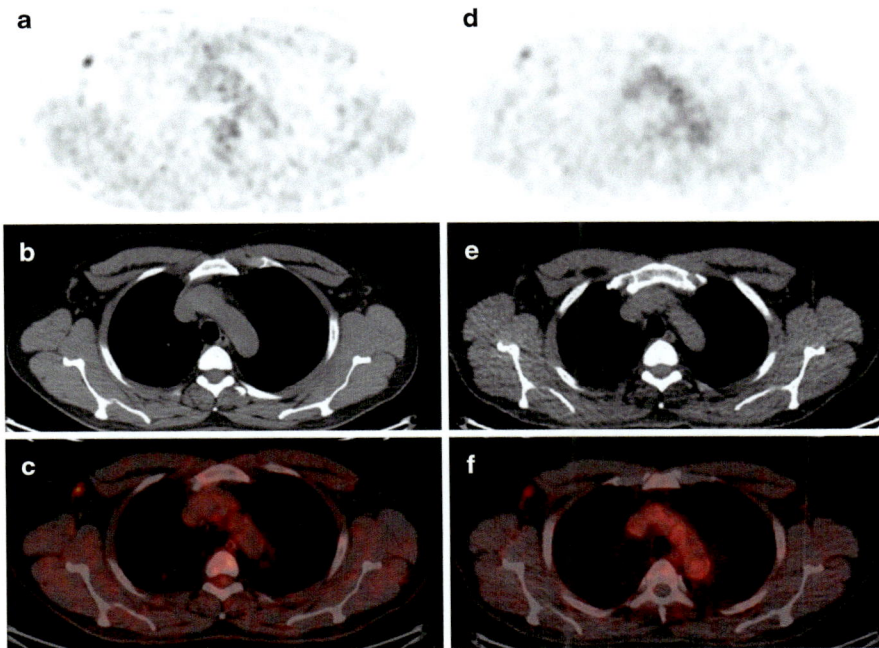

Fig. 7.3 Axial 18F-FDG PET/CT images (**a–c**) show tracer avid right level I axillary lymph node with SUVmax 5.74. Axial 68Ga-DOTAGA-IAC PET/CT images (**d–f**) show tracer avidity in the same lesion with SUVmax 2.2 (Image courtesy: Dr. Jaya Shukla)

7.1.7   Fibroblast Activating Protein Targeted Imaging

Cancer-associated fibroblasts form a major bulk of the tumor microenvironment with overexpression of fibroblast activation protein (FAP). It is also found to be overexpressed in breast cancers. Hence, FAP-specific inhibitors can be used as targeted anticancer therapy. Various 68Ga-FAP inhibitor (FAPI) PET/CT tracers have been found useful in low FDG avid breast cancers for diagnosis, staging, and can also be explored for radioligand therapy. A recent study has shown higher sensitivity of 68Ga-FAPI-04 PET/CT than FDG PET/CT for both primary and metastatic breast cancer due to its lower background activity [27]. Hence, it can play an important role in the diagnosis and staging of low FDG avid breast cancers (Fig 7.4). Radioligand therapy with FAP inhibitors for metastatic breast cancer may be useful in a patient showing avidity for FAPI-based tracers.

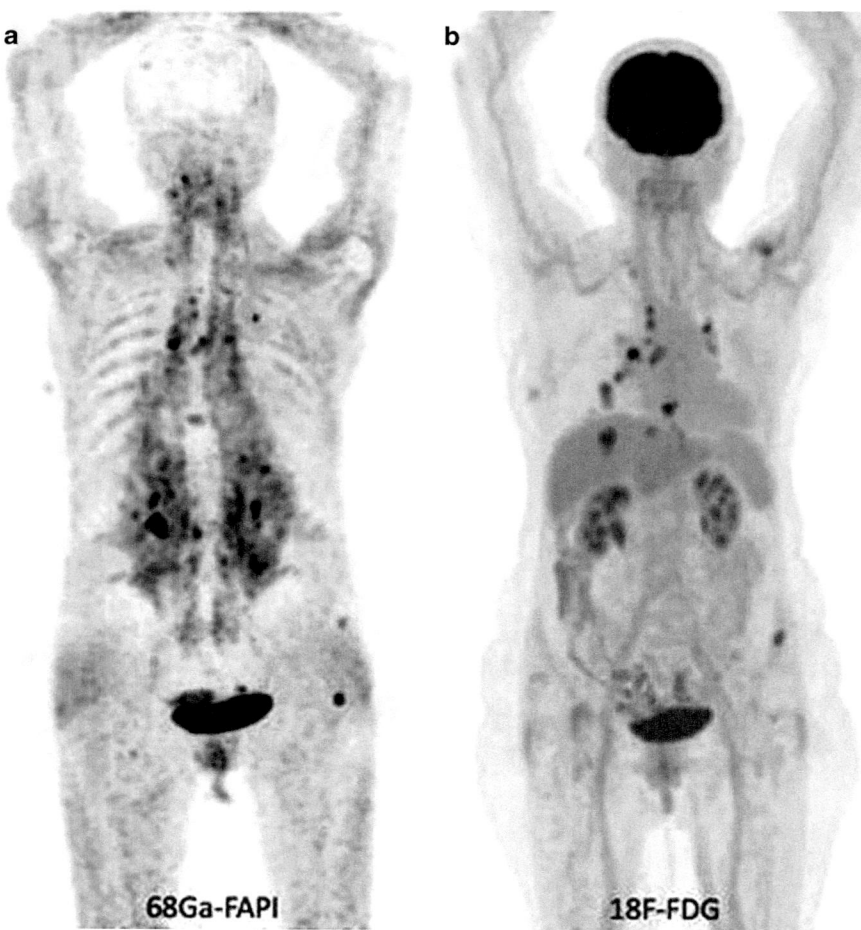

Fig. 7.4 A 76-year-old female with a history of left breast cancer (invasive lobular carcinoma), post-left modified mastectomy with axillary lymph node dissection and chemotherapy 15 years ago, referred for restaging. Ga-68 FAPI PET/CT (**a**) and FDG PET/CT (**b**) maximum intensity projection images show multiple hypermetabolic foci involving right supraclavicular, mediastinal, hilar, peri bronchial lymph nodes, left iliac crest, left transverse process of T9 and T10 vertebrae (Image courtesy: Dr. Majid Assadi)

7.1.8 Chemokine Receptor Imaging

CXCR-4 is a 7-transmembrane G-coupled receptor belonging to the chemokine receptor family and is found to be overexpressed in various tumors including breast cancer. Its activation by its endogenous ligand CXCL12, triggers tumor growth, progression, invasiveness, and metastasis [28]. Its expression is more in metastatic sites than in the primary site. CXCR4 is also expressed by the immune cells in tumor microenvironment which can be a target for immunotherapy for various cancers. Radiolabelled CXCR4-ligand for PET (68Ga-Pentixafor) has shown higher tumor accumulation, low background activity with faster clearance from non-cancer tissues. Few studies with small sample sizes have shown lower sensitivity of 68Ga-Pentixafor PET-CT than FDG PET-CT in primary and metastatic breast cancer with heterogenous avidity to various lesions (shows more avidity for invasive ductal carcinoma than lobular carcinoma and triple-negative breast cancer). There was no correlation found with the hormonal receptor positivity status on IHC. Solid tumor has shown lower CXCR4 PET avidity than FDG PET [5]. Further larger studies are needed to validate its utility in breast cancer.

7.2   PET-MRI in Breast Cancer

Early diagnosis and accurate staging of primary breast cancer is important for treatment decision making, prognostication and better treatment outcome of patients. Although, ^{18}F-FDG PET-CT has proved its efficacy in various malignancies including breast cancer, it has its limitations in the diagnosis of primary breast lesions. This is due to the variable uptake in these lesions, e.g., false negative in lobular breast cancer, ductal carcinoma in situ (DCIS), small lesions, and false positive in benign conditions like breast abscess, fibroadenomas and focal fat necrosis [29, 30]. Multiparametric Magnetic Resonance imaging (MRI) with various sequences like dynamic contrast enhanced (DCE), diffusion-weighted imaging (DWI) with apparent diffusion coefficient (ADC) mapping, and magnetic resonance spectroscopy (MRS), is a versatile tool with a better soft tissue resolution than CT. This can be useful in the diagnosis and characterization of primary breast lesion when mammography and USG findings are equivocal. MRI is also helpful in the follow-up of primary lesion after neoadjuvant or completion of chemotherapy and local radiotherapy. MRI has good sensitivity for detection of distant organ metastases like in brain and liver, especially with DWI. But there are limitations of MRI alone in the staging of breast cancer. These include its low sensitivity for detection of axillary, internal mammary lymph nodes, and lung lesions which are better detected on ^{18}F-FDG PET-CT. ^{18}F-FDG PET-CT has been commonly used for staging of advanced breast cancer (above Stage IIb), response evaluation, follow up, and detection of recurrence. But its sensitivity and specificity for detection of metastatic lesions in brain and liver are lower compared to MRI [31].

So, combined PET-MRI is being tried as a new innovation in imaging, that utilizes the advantages of both these modalities and eliminating the added radiation burden due to CT for anatomical information and attenuation correction. Solid state semiconductor PET detectors like avalanche photodiodes have made it possible to integrate PET inside the MRI gantry [32]. This allows simultaneous imaging of PET and MRI with gadolinium contrast and even dynamic imaging. MRI-based attenuation correction is done using the Dixon sequence-based segmentation method. By combining the FDG PET component with MRI increases the sensitivity and specificity of both the modalities for the diagnosis of primary tumor, its characterization, staging, follow-up, and recurrence evaluation [33, 34]. Studies have shown good correlation between FDG PET-CT metabolic parameters and findings of multiparametric MRI with histopathological ER, PR, Her-2 neu hormonal status and Ki-67 proliferation index of primary and metastatic lesions [35]. As already mentioned, FDG PET component of PET/MRI increases the sensitivity of detection of axillary, internal mammary lymph nodes and skeletal lesions whereas the MRI increases the accuracy of primary breast lesion characterization, and metastatic brain and liver lesions. PET-MRI can be very useful and versatile tool, especially for young patients requiring long-term surveillance due to less radiation burden [36]. Despite its advantages, currently PET-MRI has not gained popularity in common clinical use due to its high cost and long scan time and sometimes requiring sedation. At present, there is no data to indicate PET/MRI could replace PET/CT as the standard imaging modality for initial and subsequent therapy evaluation. Nevertheless, further studies and research are required for the evaluation of cost-effectiveness and usefulness of PET-MRI in standard clinical use.

References

1. Boers J, de Vries EF, Glaudemans AW, Hospers GA, Schröder CP. Application of PET tracers in molecular imaging for breast cancer. Curr Oncol Rep. 2020;22(8):1–6.
2. Penuelas I, Domínguez-Prado I, García-Velloso MJ, Martí-Climent JM, Rodríguez-Fraile M, Caicedo C, et al. PET tracers for clinical imaging of breast cancer. J Oncol. 2012;2012:710561.
3. Kenny L. The use of novel PET tracers to image breast cancer biologic processes such as proliferation, DNA damage and repair, and angiogenesis. J Nucl Med. 2016;57:89S–95S.
4. Kratochwil C, Flechsig P, Lindner T, Abderrahim L, Altmann A, Mier W, et al. 68Ga-FAPI PET/CT: tracer uptake in 28 different kinds of cancer. J Nucl Med. 2019;60(6):801–5.
5. Vag T, Steiger K, Rossmann A, Keller U, Noske A, Herhaus P, Ettl J, Niemeyer M, Wester HJ, Schwaiger M. PET imaging of chemokine receptor CXCR4 in patients with primary and recurrent breast carcinoma. EJNMMI Res. 2018;8(1):90.
6. Blamey RW, Hornmark-Stenstam B, Ball G, et al. ONCOPOOL: a European database for 16,944 cases of breast cancer. Eur J Cancer. 2010;46:56–71.
7. Allred DC, Harvey JM, Berardo M, Clark GM. Prognostic and predictive factors in breast cancer by immunohistochemical analysis. Mod Pathol. 1998;11:155–68.
8. DeSombre ER, Thorpe SM, Rose C, et al. Prognostic usefulness of estrogen receptor immunocytochemical assays for human breast cancer. Cancer Res. 1986;46:4256s–64s.
9. Sharangpani GM, Joshi AS, Porter K, et al. Semi-automated imaging system to quantitate estrogen and progesterone receptor immunoreactivity in human breast cancer. J Microsc. 2007;226:244–55.
10. Hammond ME, Hayes DF, Dowsett M, et al. American Society of Clinical Oncology/College of American Pathologists guideline recommendations for immunohistochemical testing of estrogen and progesterone receptors in breast cancer. J Clin Oncol. 2010;28:2784–95.
11. Hospers GA, Helmond FA, de Vries EG, Dierckx RA, de Vries EF. PET imaging of steroid receptor expression in breast and prostate cancer. Curr Pharm Des. 2008;14:3020–32.
12. McGuire AH, Dehdashti F, Siegel BA, et al. Positron tomographic assessment of 16 alpha-[18F]fluoro-17 beta-estradiol uptake in metastatic breast carcinoma. J Nucl Med. 1991;32:1526–31.
13. Peterson LM, Mankoff DA, Lawton T, et al. Quantitative imaging of estrogen receptor expression in breast cancer with PET and 18F-fluoroestradiol. J Nucl Med. 2008;49:367–74.
14. Evangelista L, Guarneri V, Conte PF. 18F-Fluoroestradiol positron emission tomography in breast cancer patients: systematic review of the literature & meta-analysis. Curr Radiopharm. 2016;9:244–57.

15. Chae SY, Ahn SH, Kim S-B, Han S, Lee SH, Oh SJ, et al. Diagnostic accuracy and safety of 16alpha-[(18)F]fluoro-17beta- oestradiol PET-CT for the assessment of oestrogen receptor status in recurrent or metastatic lesions in patients with breast cancer: a prospective cohort study. Lancet Oncol. 2019;20:546–55.
16. Arteaga CL, Sliwkowski MX, Osborne CK, et al. Treatment of HER2-positive breast cancer: current status and future perspectives. Nat Rev Clin Oncol. 2012;9(1):16–32.
17. Capala J, Bouchelouche K. Molecular imaging of HER2-positive breast cancer - a step toward an individualized "image and treat" strategy. Curr Opin Oncol. 2010;22(6):559–66.
18. Elias SG, Adams A, Wisner DJ, et al. Imaging features of HER2 overexpression in breast cancer: a systematic review and meta-analysis. Cancer Epidemiol Biomark Prev. 2014;23(8):1464–83.
19. O'Sullivan CC, Bradbury I, Campbell C, et al. Efficacy of adjuvant trastuzumab for patients with human epidermal growth factor receptor 2–positive early breast cancer and tumors ≤ 2 cm: a meta-analysis of the randomized trastuzumab trials. J Clin Oncol. 2015;33(24):2600–8.
20. Ulaner GA, Hyman D, Ross D, et al. Detection of HER2-positive metastases in patients with HER2-negative primary breast cancer using the 89Zr-DFO-trastuzumab PET/CT. J Nucl Med. 2016;57(10):1523–8.
21. Henry KE, Ulaner GA, Lewis JS. Human epidermal growth factor receptor 2-targeted PET/ single- photon emission computed tomography imaging of breast cancer: noninvasive measurement of a biomarker integral to tumor treatment and prognosis. PET Clin. 2017;12(3):269–88.
22. Vesselle H, Grierson J, Muzi M, et al. In vivo validation of 3′ deoxy-3′ -[18F]fluorothymidine ([18F]FLT) as a proliferation imaging tracer in humans: correlation of [18F]FLT uptake by positron emission tomography with Ki-67 immunohistochemistry and flow cytometry in human lung tumors. Clin Cancer Res. 2002;8(11):3315–23.
23. Kenny L, Coombes RC, Vigushin DM, Al-Nahhas A, Shousha S, Aboagye EO. Imaging early changes in proliferation at 1 week post chemotherapy: a pilot study in breast cancer patients with 3′ -deoxy-3′ -[18F]fluorothymidine positron emission tomography. Eur J Nucl Med Mol Imaging. 2007;34(9):1339–47.
24. Hussain SA, Ganesan R, Reynolds G, et al. Hypoxia-regulated carbonic anhydrase IX expression is associated with poor survival in patients with invasive breast cancer. Br J Cancer. 2007;96(1):104–9.
25. Beer AJ, Niemeyer M, Carlsen J, et al. Patterns of αvβ3 expression in primary and metastatic human breast cancer as shown by 18F-galacto-RGD PET. J Nucl Med. 2008;49(2):255–9.
26. Ming Y, Wu N, Qian T, Li X, Wan DQ, Li C, Li Y, Wu Z, Wang X, Liu J, Wu N. Progress and future trends in PET/CT and PET/MRI molecular imaging approaches for breast cancer. Front Oncol. 2020;12(10):1301.
27. Kömek H, Can C, Güzel Y, Oruç Z, Gündoğan C, Yildirim ÖA, Kaplan İ, Erdur E, Yıldırım MS, Çakabay B. 68Ga-FAPI-04 PET/CT, a new step in breast cancer imaging: a comparative pilot study with the 18F-FDG PET/CT. Ann Nucl Med. 2021;35:744–52.
28. Zlotnik A. Chemokines and cancer. Int J Cancer. 2006;119:2026–9.
29. Bos R, van Der Hoeven JJ, van Der Wall E, et al. Biologic correlates of (18) fluorodeoxyglucose uptake in human breast cancer measured by positron emission tomography. J Clin Oncol. 2002;20:379–87.
30. Kim MY, Cho N, Chang JM, Yun BL, Bae MS, Kang KW, Moon WK. Mammography and ultrasonography evaluation of unexpected focal 18F-FDG uptakes in breast on PET/CT. Acta Radiol. 2012;53(3):249–54.
31. Pujara AC, Kim E, Axelrod D, Melsaether AN. PET/MRI in breast cancer. J Magn Reson Imaging. 2019;49(2):328–42.
32. Aklan B, Paulus DH, Fual D, Geppert C, Sigmund EE, Melsaether A, Wenkel E, Braun H, Ziegler S, Quick HH. Towards simultaneous PET/MR breast imaging: systematic evaluation and integration of an RF breast coil. In: International society for magnetic resonance in medicine, 21st annual meeting & exhibition 2013 Apr, pp. 22–26.
33. Garcia-Velloso MJ, Ribelles MJ, Rodriguez M, Fernandez-Montero A, Sancho L, Prieto E, Santisteban M, Rodriguez-Spiteri N, Idoate MA, Martinez-Regueira F, Elizalde A. MRI fused with prone FDG PET/CT improves the primary tumour staging of patients with breast cancer. Eur Radiol. 2017;27(8):3190–8.

34. Domingues RC, Carneiro MP, Lopes FC, Domingues RC, da Fonseca LM, Gasparetto EL. Whole-body MRI and FDG PET fused images for evaluation of patients with cancer. Am J Roentgenol. 2009;192(4):1012–20.
35. Baba S, Isoda T, Maruoka Y, Kitamura Y, Sasaki M, Yoshida T, Honda H. Diagnostic and prognostic value of pretreatment SUV in 18F-FDG/PET in breast cancer: comparison with apparent diffusion coefficient from diffusion-weighted MR imaging. J Nucl Med. 2014;55(5):736–42.
36. Melsaether AN, Raad RA, Pujara AC, Ponzo FD, Pysarenko KM, Jhaveri K, Babb JS, Sigmund EE, Kim SG, Moy LA. Comparison of whole-body 18F FDG PET/MR imaging and whole-body 18F FDG PET/CT in terms of lesion detection and radiation dose in patients with breast cancer. Radiology. 2016;281(1):193–202.

Clinical Cases

8

Narainder K. Gupta, Kanhaiyalal Agrawal, and Bhagwant Rai Mittal

Contents

N. K. Gupta
Department of Radiology, Hospital of the University of Pennsylvania, Philadelphia, PA, USA
e-mail: Narainder.Gupta@pennmedicine.upenn.edu

K. Agrawal (✉)
Department of Nuclear Medicine, AIIMS, Bhubaneswar, India

B. R. Mittal
Department of Nuclear Medicine, PGIMER, Chandigarh, India

© The Author(s), under exclusive license to Springer Nature Switzerland AG 2023
R. Kumar et al. (eds.), *PET/CT in Breast Cancer*, Clinicians' Guides to
Radionuclide Hybrid Imaging, https://doi.org/10.1007/978-3-031-29590-4_8

8.1   Case-1: FDG PET-CT in Staging of Breast Cancer

Clinical Details A 49-year-old lady with left breast carcinoma (invasive ductal carcinoma non-specific type poorly differentiated) underwent left modified radical mastectomy and axillary clearance (Fig. 8.1).

Teaching Points
FDG PET/CT is a sensitive and specific imaging modality for identifying distant metastases in patients with breast cancer missed by or indeterminate on conventional imaging.

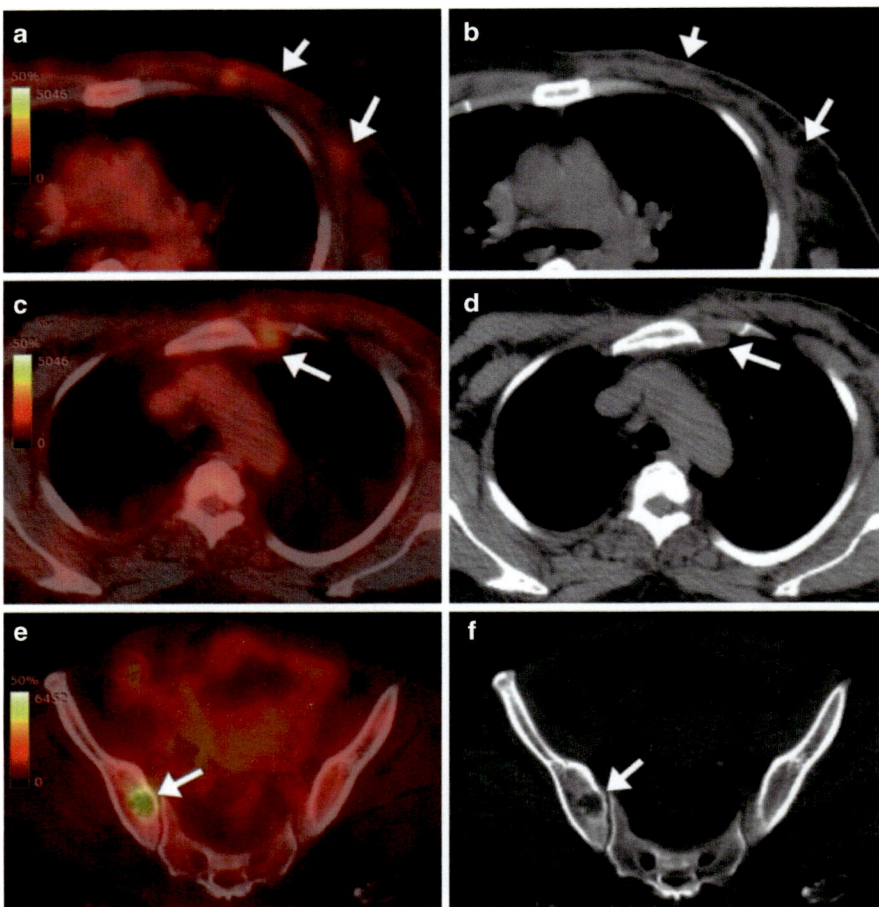

Fig. 8.1 FDG PET-CT shows minimally hypermetabolic fibrotic changes in the left anterior chest wall suggestive of post-surgical inflammation (arrows in **a**, **b**), prominent left internal mammary lymph node showing increased tracer uptake (arrows in **c**, **d**) and an FDG avid lytic lesion in the right iliac bone suggestive of solitary bone metastatic disease (arrows in **e**, **f**)

8.2   Case-2: Multifocal Primary Disease

Clinical Details 76-year-old lady with biopsy-proven case of carcinoma right breast underwent FDG PET-CT for staging (Fig. 8.2).

Teaching Points
FDG PET-CT frequently detects multiple foci of disease in the breast.

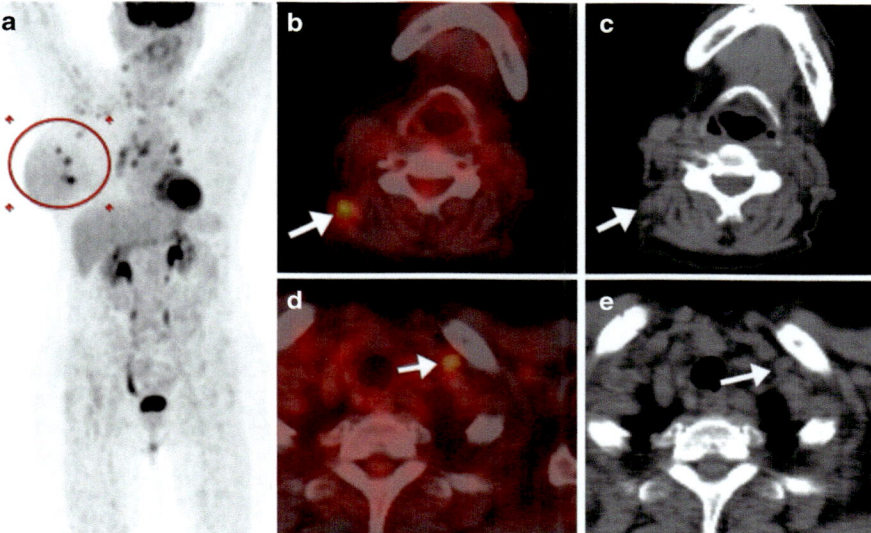

Fig. 8.2 (**A**) FDG PET-CT shows multiple foci of increased tracer uptake in the right breast with right axillary and mediastinal lymph nodes uptake in the MIP image (a). Axial PET-CT and CT images show hypermetabolic right level V and left supraclavicular lymph nodes suggestive of metastatic disease (arrows in b–e). (**B**) Axial section through the right breast shows multiple foci of increased tracer uptake in the right breast parenchyma suggestive of multifocal primary disease (arrows a–f)

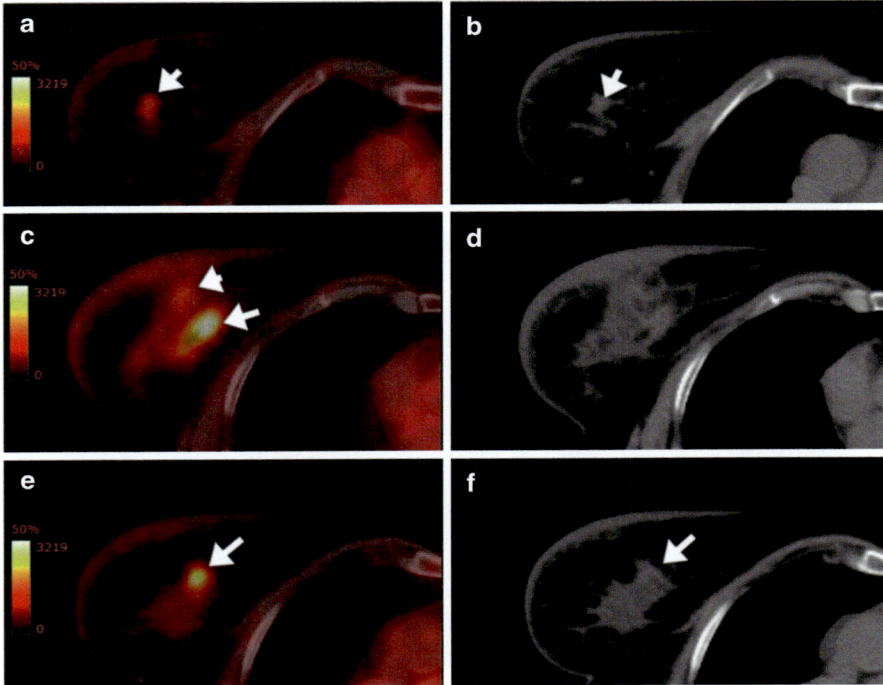

Fig. 8.2 (continued)

8.3   Case-3: False Positives on FDG PET-CT

Clinical Details A 73-year-old female with biopsy-proven moderately differentiated invasive ductal carcinoma NOS subtype underwent FDG PET-CT for staging (Fig. 8.3).

Teaching Point
False positive uptake may be seen in lung inflammation/infection and degenerative changes in bones.

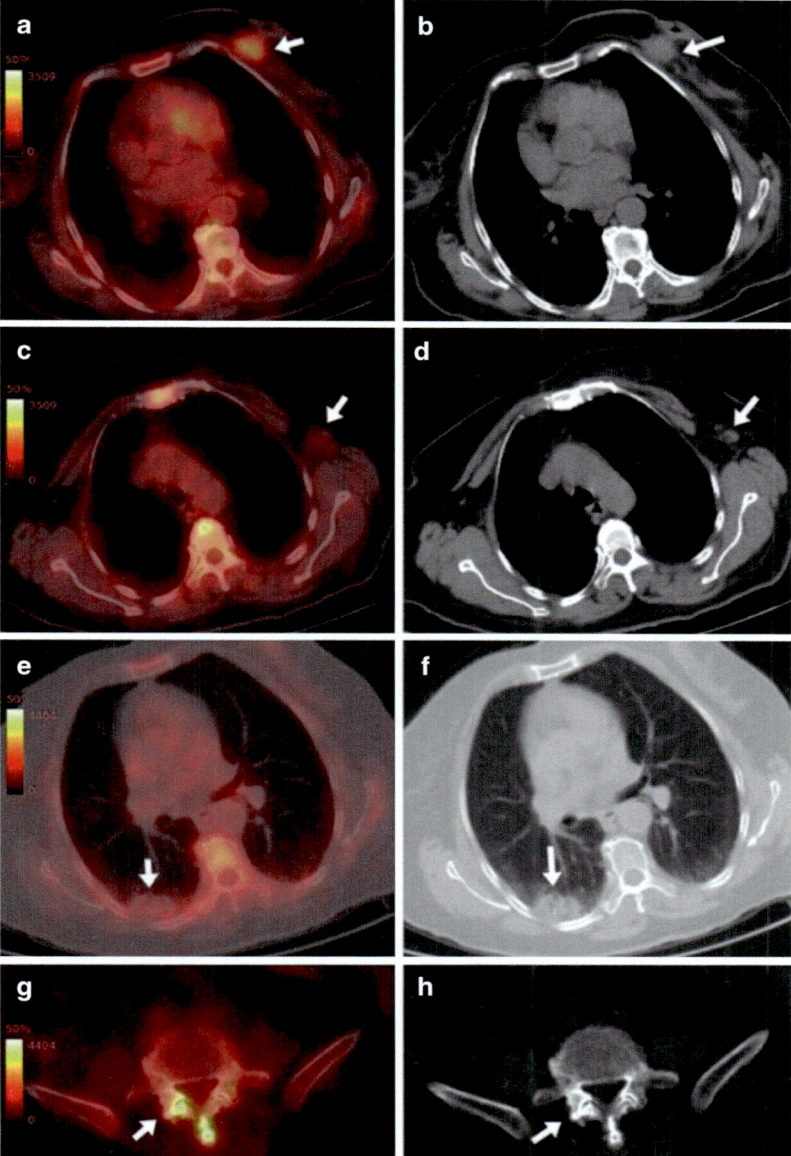

Fig. 8.3 (**a, b**) Hypermetabolic irregular soft tissue density lesion in the retroareolar region of the left breast with SUVmax 7.8 suggestive of primary malignant lesion (arrows). The lesion is seen in continuation with the nipple anteriorly and loss of fat plane with the pectoralis muscle. (**c, d**) Mildly hypermetabolic subcentimeter left axillary lymph nodes with SUVmax 3.1 (arrows) could be metastatic. (**e, f**) Minimally hypermetabolic consolidatory mass in the right lower lobe lung posteriorly (arrows) is mostly inflammatory aspect. (**g, h**) Mild uptake is seen at the right L3-4 facet joint showing degenerative changes (arrows) suggestive of facetal arthropathy

8.4   Case-4: False-Positive PET-CT Due to Fat Necrosis

Clinical Details A 62-year-old female patient, with a history of right breast cancer in 2000 status post lumpectomy and radiation. In 2015, the patient was found to have right breast intra-ductal carcinoma and is now status post-bilateral mastectomy with free flap reconstruction in March 2015. Patient was on chemotherapy at this time for metastatic carcinoma and was being followed with PET-CT scan (Fig. 8.4).

Teaching Points
1. On PET-CT, the fat necrosis can cause false-positive scan for malignancy and there can be moderate to intense FDG uptake in fat necrosis. This uptake can persist for a long time.
2. Ultrasound can be useful to evaluate fat necrosis but it cannot always distinguish fat necrosis from malignancy and therefore biopsy is required in certain cases. Ultrasound in these cases should be interpreted in the context of mammographic findings.

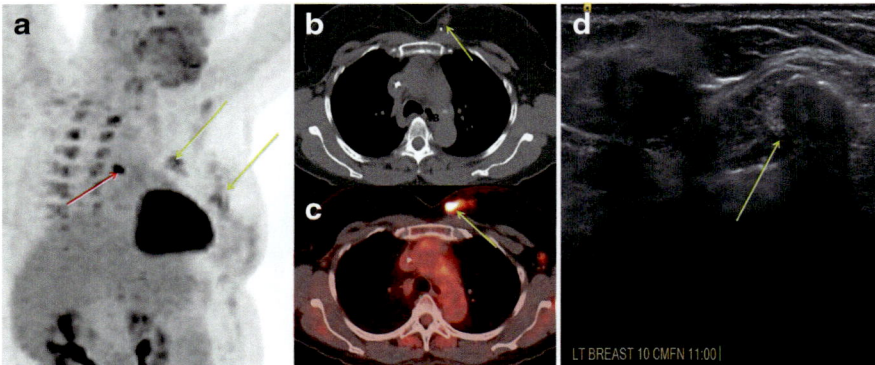

Fig. 8.4 Maximum intensity projection FDG PET-CT image (**a**) showing two foci of tracer uptake in the left breast (yellow arrows) and right hilar lymph node (red arrow). Trans-axial fused PET-CT image (**c**) shows the superior focus of tracer uptake within left reconstructed breast and a clear focus of fat is noticed within this lesion on CT slice (**b**). However, ultrasound was not able to distinguish fat necrosis from malignancy (**d**). In this case both FDG avid lesions were biopsied proven fat necrosis

8.5   Case-5: False Positive Uptake in the Lactating Breasts

Clinical Details   A 36-year-old female with a history of multiple melanomas and in 2014, a very concerning in-transit metastatic focus is seen in her left thigh. She was breast-feeding her first baby in October, 2014. A staging PET-CT scan at that time was abnormal for a focal area of increased tracer uptake in the left medial thigh that was later proven to be an in-transit metastatic lesion. She had almost bilateral symmetrical moderate FDG activity in her breasts due to lactation. On a subsequent staging PET-CT scan in April 2015, the lactating breast activity got normalized. She got pregnant again against oncology advice and again lactating at the time of PET-CT scan in August 2016 (Fig. 8.5

Teaching Points
1. Uptake of FDG in breasts is related to infant feeding and can be asymmetric or unilateral depending upon feeding habits.
2. Unilateral breast uptake should include differential diagnosis of infection, radiation, lactation, breast carcinoma, and lymphoma, and further clinical correlation is usually required. If warranted, mammograms and ultrasounds should be performed.

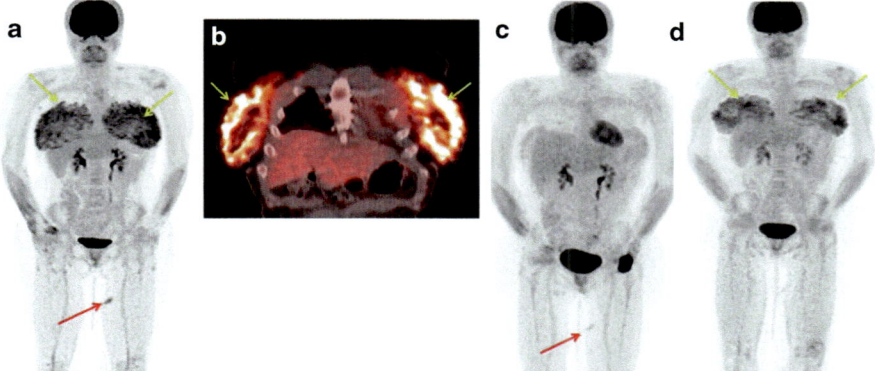

Fig. 8.5   Maximum intensity projection image (**a**) and coronal fused image (**b**) from a FDG PET-CT scan showing moderate FDG uptake in the lactating breasts (yellow arrows) and a focal uptake (red arrow) highly suspicious of in-transit metastatic lesion. The uptake in breasts is normalized (**c**), however, uptake is again seen in both breasts (arrows) on the scan after a few months of the birth of a second child. (**d**) The in-transit focus has resolved on treatment

8.6   Case-6: False Positive in Fibroadenoma

Clinical Details A 22-year-old female with stage IIB bulky Hodgkin's lymphoma with extranodal involvement and PET-CT was done for restaging. She was started on ABVD in February 2017. She achieved metabolic CR after cycle 2 and continued to be in CR after cycle 4B and after 6B (her last chemotherapy was in July 2017). She completed consolidative RT in September 2017 (Fig. 8.6).

Teaching Points
1. Fibroadenomas may show uptake and may be confusing in patients with systemic malignancy. PET-CT can help differentiate by showing differential uptake as in this case.
2. Fibroadenomas are the most common benign breast lesions in reproductive-age females.

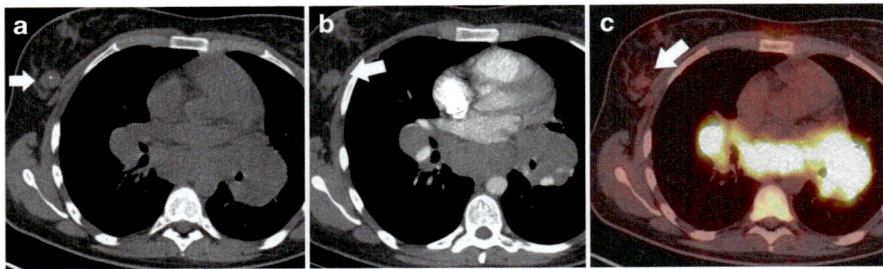

Fig. 8.6 Plain CT scan (**a**) showing right breast well-defined lesion (arrow) with calcific fleck. On CECT image (**b**), she had homogenous mildly enhancing mediastinal lymphadenopathy and non-enhancing soft tissue nodule in the right breast (arrow). Fused axial FDG PET-CT image (**c**) shows significant uptake in mediastinal lymphadenopathy. However, there is comparatively minimal uptake in the right breast lesion (arrow). The lesion was proved to be fibroadenoma

8.7 Case-7: False-Negative FDG PET-CT in Lobular Carcinoma

Clinical Details A 45-year-old lady with moderately differentiated invasive lobular carcinoma of the right breast underwent FDG PET-CT for staging (Fig. 8.7).

Teaching Point

Lobular carcinoma may not show FDG avidity. Sentinel node biopsy should be advised to rule out metastatic disease in ipsilateral FDG non-avid lymph nodes.

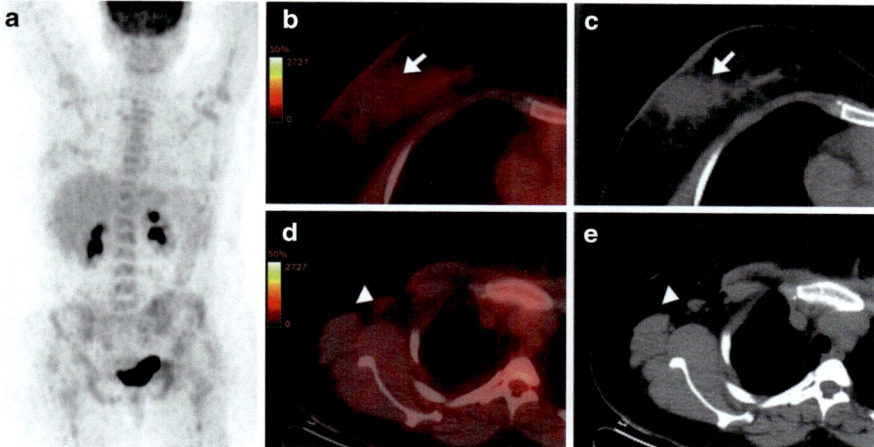

Fig. 8.7 MIP FDG PET-CT (**a**) shows no significant tracer uptake in the irregular soft tissue mass measuring 3 cm in the right breast with SUVmax 0.79 (arrows in **b**, **c**). No significant tracer uptake is seen in subcentimeter right axillary lymph node with SUVmax 0.72 with thick cortex although there is preserved fat hilum

8.8   Case-8: Paget's Disease of Breast

Clinical Details A 48-year-female patient is status post left lumpectomy for an unknown pathology and radiation in 2000. Patient reported with 2 months of breast stiffness and infection on the left (Fig. 8.8).

Teaching Points
1. Paget's disease presents with eczema and imaging plays a role to evaluate extent of disease.
2. Mammogram and Ultrasound may be normal in such patients and MR imaging may be helpful.
3. Sometimes scar tissue may show more avid uptake than primary malignancy.

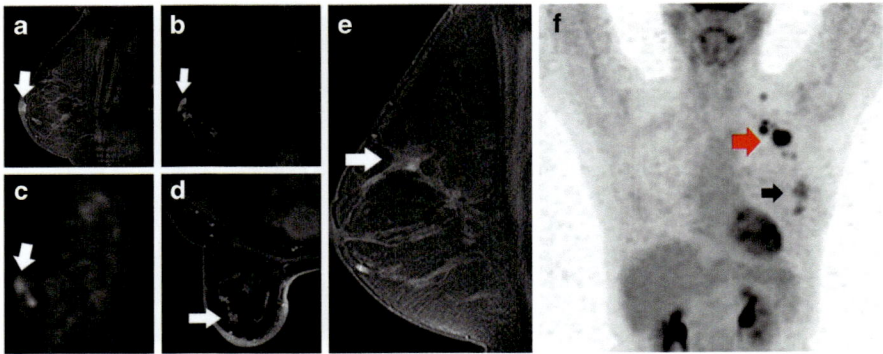

Fig. 8.8 Left breast MR images T2 Fat sat (**a**), subtraction images (**b, c**) show moderate enhancement posterior to the nipple and extending to the nipple and skin (arrows) consistent with Paget's disease of the breast. MR images T2 weighted (**d**) and Fatsat (**e**) show the non-enhancing scar with fat necrosis (arrows) consistent with post-lumpectomy status. FDG PET-CT maximum intensity image (**f**) showing uptake in the scar (red arrow) and near the lesion (black arrow)

8.9 Case-9: Role of FDG PET-CT in Indeterminate Lesions on CT

Clinical Details A 83-year-old lady presented with right axillary lymphadenopathy, which on excision biopsy showed metastatic adenocarcinoma mostly of breast origin. However, mammogram and USG of the right breast did not show evidence of carcinoma in the right breast. FDG PET-CT was performed for further assessment (Fig. 8.9).

Teaching Points
1. CT studies sometimes show suspicious lesions when performed for metastatic assessment. FDG PET-CT is specific in characterizing most of these lesions and helps in better patient management.

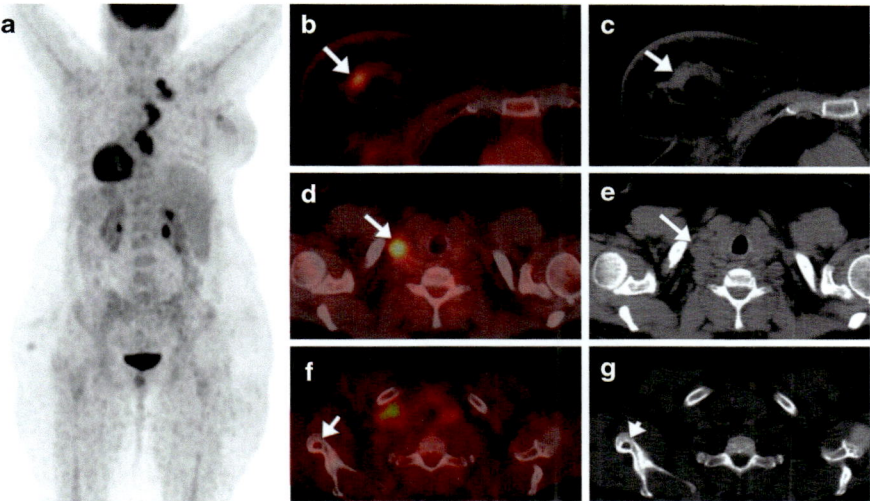

Fig. 8.9 FDG PET-CT (A-MIP) shows intense tracer uptake in the midline in the thorax with minimal tracer uptake in the right breast. Axial PET-CT and CT images show mild focal hypermetabolism in the right breast parenchyma (arrows in **b, c**) suggestive of primary malignant lesion. Intensely hypermetabolic metastatic right supraclavicular (arrows in **d, e**) and mediastinal lymph nodes are seen. Further, metabolically inactive lucency is seen in the right scapula (arrows in **f, g**) indicative of benign pathology. FDG PET-CT helps in ruling out metastatic disease in indeterminate lesions on anatomical lesion

8.10 Case-10: Role of FDG PET-CT in Indeterminate Lesions on CT

Clinical Details A 48-year-old lady with moderately differentiated invasive ductal carcinoma (NOS) of the right breast underwent breast conservative surgery. Restaging FDG PET-CT was performed (Fig. 8.10).

Teaching points
1. Metastatic pulmonary nodules more than 8 mm in size usually show increased FDG uptake.
2. Small lung nodules less than 8 mm may be false negative on FDG PET and follow-up imaging should be indicated.

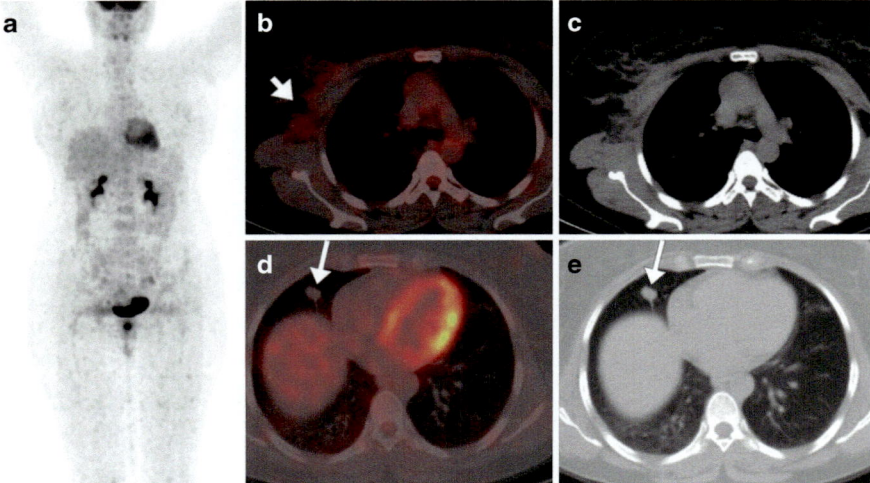

Fig. 8.10 FDG PET-CT (MIP–a) shows minimally hypermetabolic fibrotic changes in the right breast suggestive of post-surgical changes (arrow in **b**, **c**). There is a metabolically inactive 11 mm soft tissue nodule in the right lung middle lobe likely a benign nodule (arrows in **d**, **e**). On follow up CT, there was no interval change in size of the nodule confirming the benign aspect

8.11 Case-11: Indeterminate Lesions on FDG PET-CT

Clinical Details A 62-year-old lady with poorly differentiated invasive left mammary carcinoma with ductal and lobular features underwent left modified radical mastectomy and axillary clearance. FDG PET-CT was performed 10 days post-surgery as a part of metastatic assessment (Fig. 8.11).

Teaching Points
1. FDG PET-CT is helpful in staging of the breast carcinoma by ruling out metastasis in the benign lesions.
2. Post-operative changes may be seen early after surgery and should be reported cautiously.
3. Small lung nodules less than 8 mm may be false negative on FDG PET and follow-up imaging should be indicated.

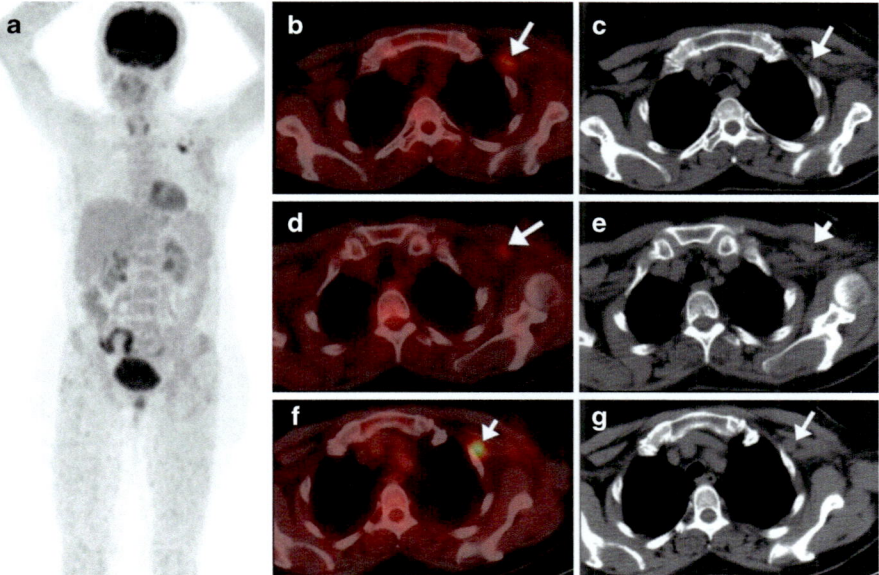

Fig. 8.11 (**A**) Restaging FDG PET-CT (a—MIP image) shows low-grade hypermetabolic sub-centimeter left interpectoral and subpectoral lymph nodes (arrows in b–g) suggestive of metastatic disease

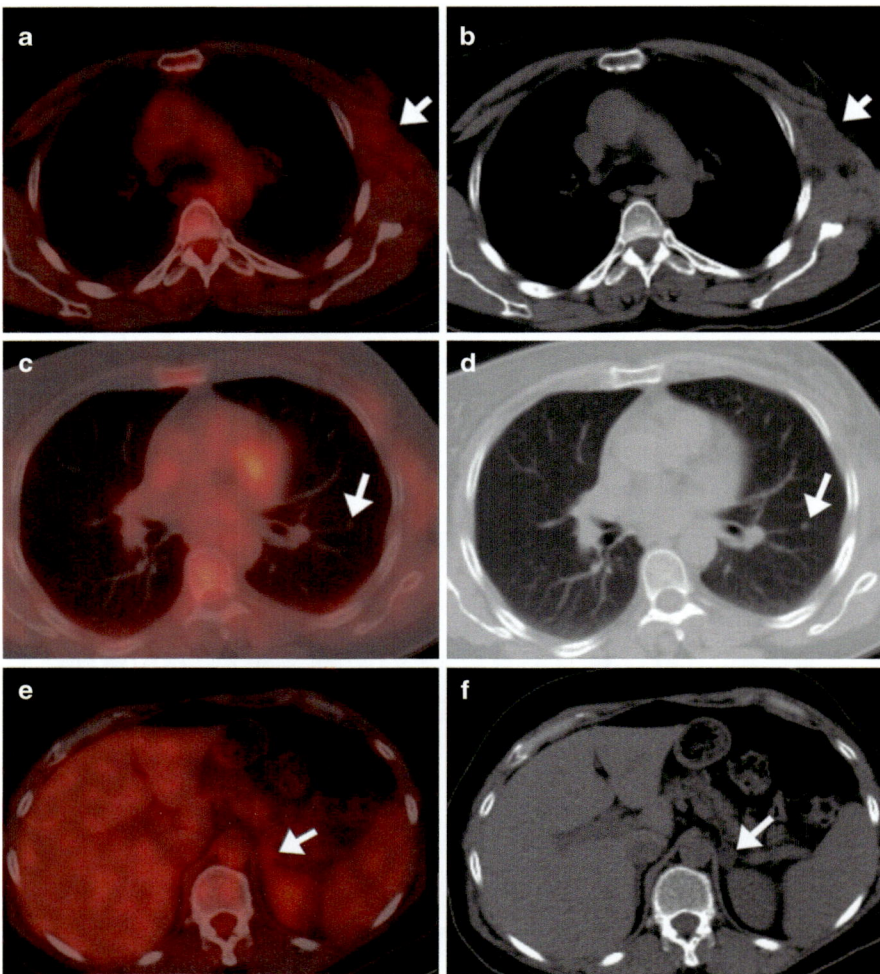

Fig. 8.11 (**B**) Axial fused PET-CT and CT images show minimally hypermetabolic thin-walled cystic lesion in the left axilla suggestive of post-operative seroma (arrows in **a, b**). No uptake is seen in the 4-mm nodule in the left lower lobe lung (arrows in **c, d**) which is indeterminate on PET as the size of nodule is below the resolution of PET scanner. Metabolically inactive nodule is seen in the left adrenal gland suggestive of an adenoma (arrows in **e, f**)

8.12   Case-12: Recurrent Disease

Clinical Details   A 42-year-old lady with a history of right breast carcinoma, post right mastectomy, and axillary clearance. Histopathology showed ductal carcinoma in situ. She presented with right anterior wall chest nodules after 14 months of the treatment (Fig. 8.12).

Teaching Point
1. FDG PET-CT detects disease recurrence early in the course of the disease.

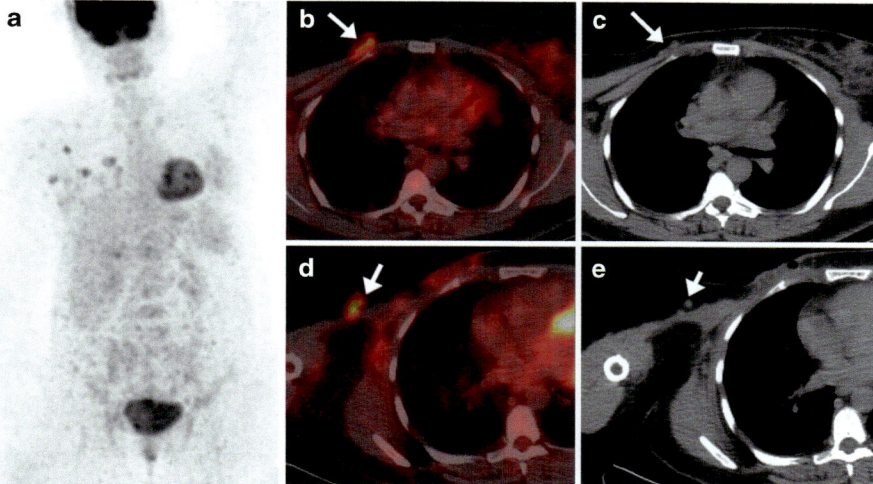

Fig. 8.12 FDG PET-CT shows focal increased tracer uptake in the right chest wall on MIP image (**a**), which on axial CT and PET-CT images (**b–e**) shows hypermetabolic subcentimeter right anterior chest wall nodules (arrows). Histopathology from the nodules revealed recurrent high-grade invasive ductal carcinoma, NOS

8.13   Case-13: FDG PET-CT in Response Assessment

Clinical Details A 41-year-old gentleman with left breast carcinoma, post lumpectomy and chemotherapy. The patient was on immunotherapy. FDG PET-CT was at baseline and post-treatment to evaluate treatment response (Fig. 8.13).

Teaching Points
1. FDG PET-CT detects early progression compared to anatomical imaging.
2. In this case, there is metabolically progression in the bone lesion but no significant changes are seen on CT.

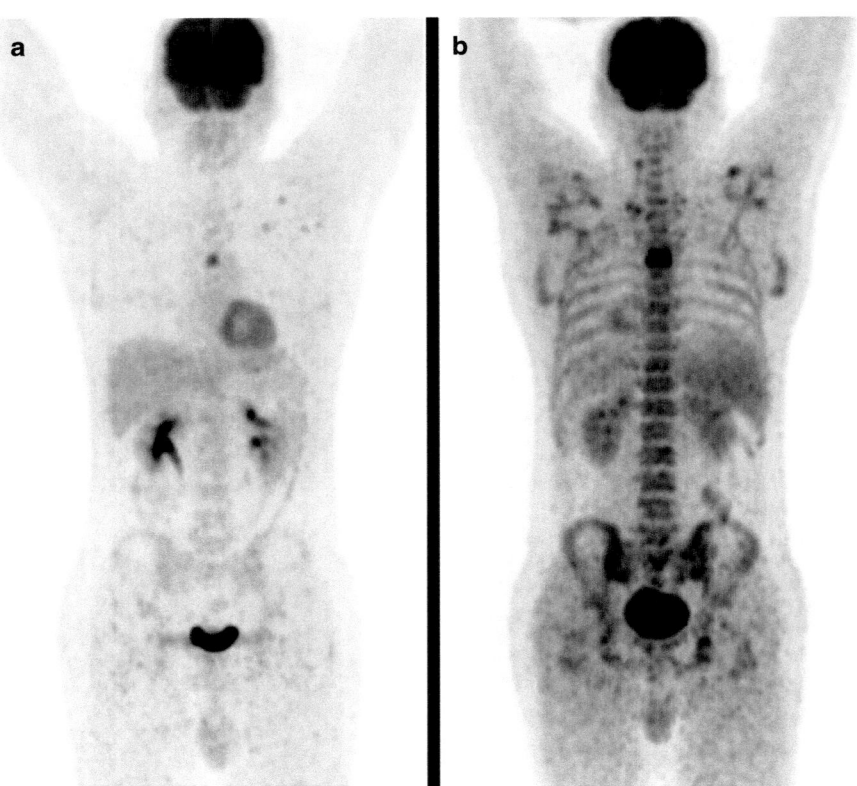

Fig. 8.13 (A) FDG PET-CT MIP images at baseline (a) and post-treatment (b) showing increased tracer uptake in dorsal vertebra in the post-treatment image

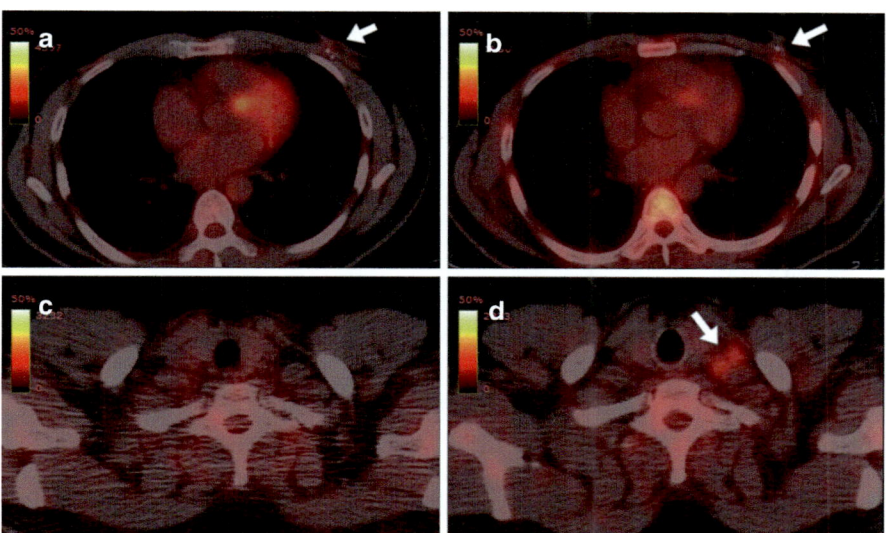

Fig. 8.13 (**B**) Axial images show post-surgical changes in the left anterior chest wall (arrows in **a**, **b**). There are interval of new hypermetabolic metastatic left supraclavicular lymph nodes (arrow in **d**) on post-therapy scan compared to baseline scan (**c**)

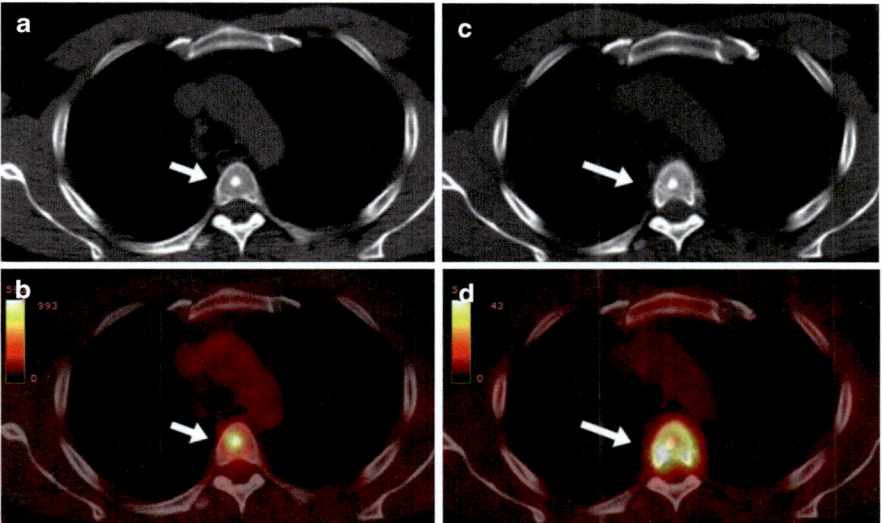

Fig. 8.13 (**C**) Axial images at D4 vertebral level show FDG avid focal sclerosis in the D4 vertebral body and SUVmax 6.4 (arrows in **a**, **b**) at baseline scan, which shows no significant change in posttreatment CT (arrow in **c**), however, post-treatment PET shows an increase in FDG avidity of the lesion with SUVmax 11.9 suggestive of disease progression

8.14   Case-14: FDG PET-CT in Response Assessment

Clinical Details A 57-year-old lady with carcinoma right breast underwent FDG PET-CT for treatment response assessment after chemotherapy (Fig. 8.14).

Moreover, anatomically patient had stable disease, however, PET shows partial treatment response.

Teaching Points
1. FDG PET-CT shows early treatment changes compared to anatomical imaging.
2. In this case, there is metabolically regression in disease but size of lesions is stable.
3. FDG PET-CT is helpful in better treatment response assessment in metastatic breast cancer compared to anatomical imaging.

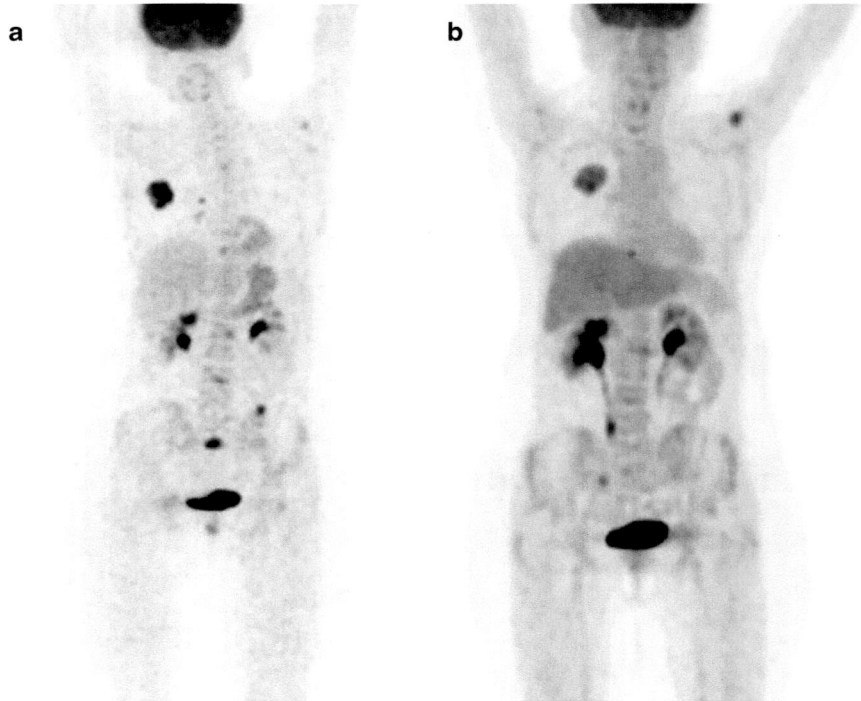

Fig. 8.14 (**A**) (a) represents maximum intensity projection (MIP) FDG PET image at baseline; (b) represents FDG PET MIP image post-chemotherapy

BASELINE **POST-TREATMENT**

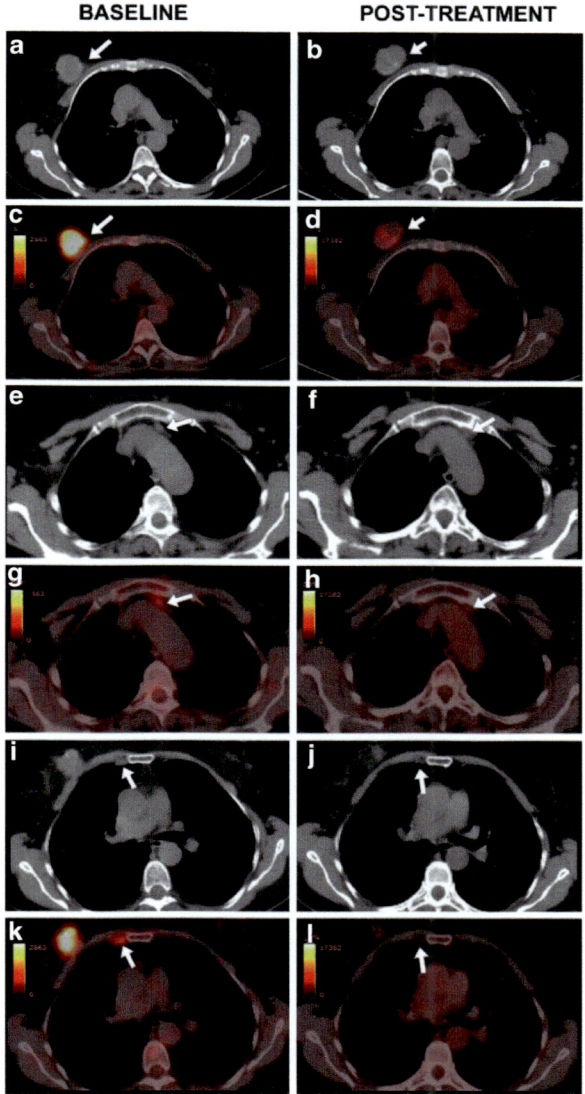

Fig. 8.14 (**B**) (a–d) axial CT and fused PET-CT images at baseline show intensely hypermetabolic irregular soft tissue density mass lesion with specs of calcification in the upper inner quadrant of the right breast measuring 34 × 29 mm and SUVmax 13.4 (arrows). Post-treatment images on the right-side show interval increase in size but regression in metabolic activity of the lesion measuring 42 × 31 mm and SUVmax 5.3 (arrows). Although there is anatomically stable disease, there is partial metabolic response. (e–h) axial CT and fused PET-CT images at baseline show subcentimeter metastatic prevascular lymph node measuring 6 mm in SAD with SUVmax 2.1 (arrows). Post-treatment images on the right-side show interval of no significant change in size measuring 5 mm, however, there is resolution of metabolic activity (arrows). (i–l) axial CT and fused PET-CT images at baseline show subcentimeter metastatic right internal mammary lymph node measuring 8 mm in SAD and SUVmax 2.1 (arrows). Post-treatment images on the right-side show interval regression in size and complete resolution of metabolic activity (arrows)

BASELINE   **POST-TREATMENT**

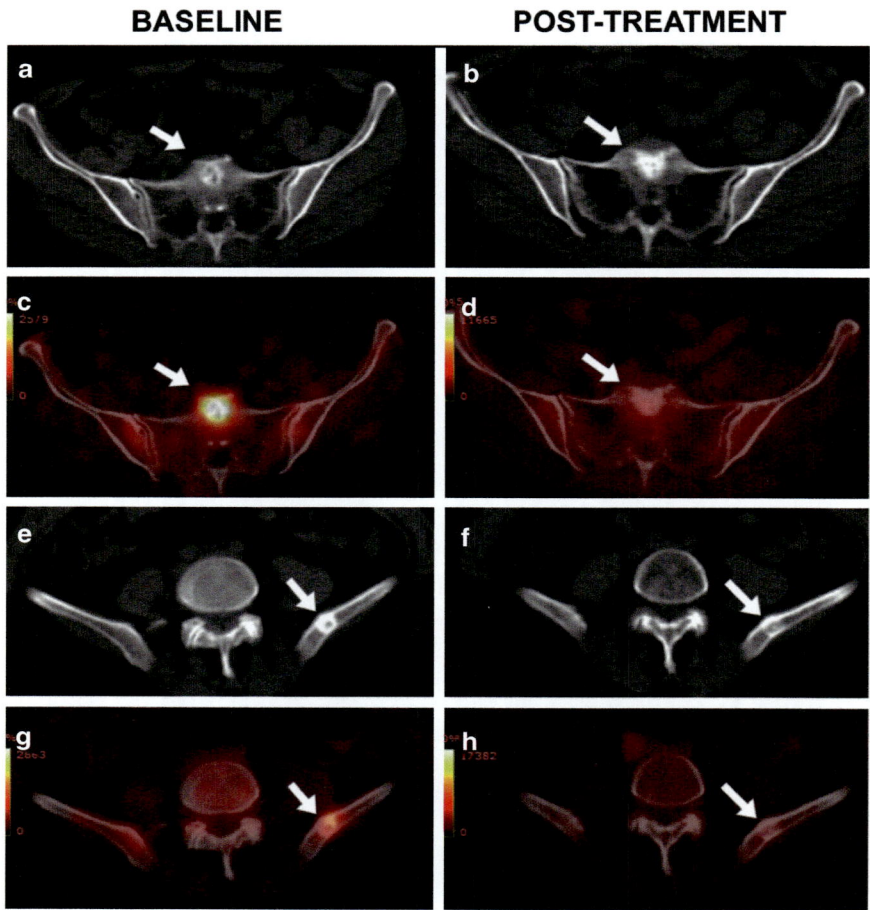

Fig. 8.14 (**C**): (a, c, e, g) Axial CT and fused PET-CT images at baseline on the left side show hypermetabolic sclerotic lesions in the sacrum and left iliac bone (arrows). (b, d, f, h) axial CT and fused PET-CT images post-chemotherapy show significant regression in metabolic activity (arrows) with increase in sclerosis in sacral lesion but no significant change in left iliac bone lesion